Going! Going! Going! Goooone Nuts

A Nutritional Journey for a Healthy Life

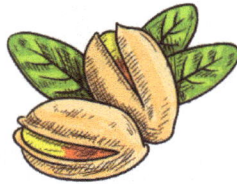

Halsey Cruickshank

ISBN: 979-8-9888447-2-3

Table of Contents

Introduction
Nuts - Nourishing Treasures from the Plant Kingdom *1*

Chapter One
Nuts - Secret Versatile Treasures *4*

Chapter Two
Almond - Wholesome Nut *13*

Chapter Three
Brazil Nut - Bountiful Nut *17*

Chapter Four
Cashew - Buttery Nut *21*

Chapter Five
Chestnut - Wholesome Nut *25*

Chapter Six
Horse Chestnut – Revitalizing Nut *29*

Chapter Seven
Coconut – Tropical Re-freshness *32*

Chapter Eight
Hazelnuts – Irresistible Nut *41*

Chapter Nine
Macadamia – Luxurious Nut *44*

Chapter Ten
Pecan – Decadent Nut *48*

Chapter Eleven
Penuts - Nutrilicious Nut..*51*

Chapter Twelve
Pine Nut — Elevator Nut..*56*

Chapter Thirteen
Pistachio - Vibrant Nut...*59*

Chapter Fourteen
Walnuts — Natural Goodness.................................*63*

Chapter Fifteen
Continental Nuts: Global Delights........................*67*

About the Author
Author Bio: Halsey Cruickshank............................*108*

Introduction

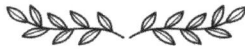

Nuts - Nourishing Treasures from the Plant Kingdom

Nuts are a delicious, nutritious, and versatile food that has been enjoyed by people around the world for centuries. From almonds and walnuts to cashews and pistachios, each variety offers a unique taste and a wealth of health benefits. Nuts are a pantry staple that can be enjoyed as a snack, incorporated into recipes, or used to make nut butters and oils. Whether you're a seasoned nut enthusiast or just discovering the world of nuts, there's something for everyone to love about these crunchy and flavorful treats.

History of Nuts in Cultures

Nuts have played a significant role in the history and culture of various civilizations across the globe. Here are a few examples:

- In ancient Greece and Rome, nuts were highly valued for their culinary and medicinal properties. Almonds, olives, and walnuts were particularly popular, and they were often used in religious ceremonies and offerings to deities.

- Native American cultures in the southwestern United States and Mexico relied heavily on pinon pine nuts as a source of food and sustenance. These nuts were stored for use throughout the year and incorporated into traditional dishes, ceremonial practices, and medicinal remedies.

- Pistachios and almonds hold a special place in Middle Eastern cuisine. In Iran, pistachios are a common ingredient in sweets, desserts, and traditional Persian ice cream. Their vibrant green color and nutty flavor add a touch of elegance and sophistication to various dishes.

- Walnuts and chestnuts hold deep cultural significance in China. Walnuts are believed to promote brain health and longevity, while chestnuts are often used to treat digestive issues and are a popular winter delicacy.

- In European regions, particularly Italy and France, chestnuts have been a staple food for centuries. They are often roasted and enjoyed as a snack or incorporated into savory dishes like soups and stuffing.

- Nuts have also played a prominent role in African cultures for generations. Shea nuts, native to West Africa, have been valued for their medicinal properties and as a source of food and fuel. Kola nuts, also native to Africa, are considered symbols of hospitality and friendship and are often used in traditional ceremonies and rituals.

The rich history of nuts across various cultures highlights their enduring importance as a source of nutrition, flavor, and cultural significance. Their versatility and adaptability have made them a treasured ingredient in cuisines worldwide.

A Culinary Delight

Nuts offer a culinary versatility that makes them a welcome addition to any kitchen. Their crunchy texture and rich flavor complement a wide range of dishes, from salads and soups to main courses and desserts. Nuts can be enjoyed raw, roasted, or ground, and they can be used to make nut butter, oils, and flour.

Nutritional Powerhouse

Beyond their culinary appeal, nuts are packed with essential nutrients that support overall health and well-being. They are a rich source of protein, fiber, healthy fats, vitamins, and minerals. These nutrients contribute to various health benefits, including:

- Improved heart health

- Reduced risk of chronic diseases

- Enhanced cognitive function

- Weight management

- Stronger bones

Conclusion

Nuts are a delicious, nutritious, and versatile food that has been cherished for centuries. Their rich history, culinary adaptability, and abundance of health benefits make them a valuable addition to any diet. Whether you're snacking on them on the go, incorporating them into your culinary creations, or enjoying their health-promoting properties, nuts are a true gift from nature.

Chapter One

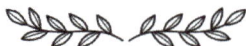

Nuts - Secret Versatile Treasures

N ature has provided us with an abundance of nutritious and delicious foods, and nuts stand out as "Flavorful delights that tantalize the taste buds". These versatile treats, packed with essential nutrients and flavor, have been enjoyed by people around the world for centuries. From the familiar crunch of almonds and walnuts to the buttery smoothness of cashews and pistachios, each type of nut offers a unique culinary experience and a wealth of health benefits.

Nuts: A Culinary Adventure

Nuts are not just a tasty snack; they are culinary chameleons that seamlessly blend into a wide range of dishes. Their crunchy texture and rich flavor complement a variety of cuisines, adding depth and complexity to both sweet and savory creations. Whether you're sprinkling them over salads for a burst of crunch, incorporating them into hearty soups and stews for added richness, or using them to craft decadent desserts, nuts are a versatile ingredient that can elevate any dish.

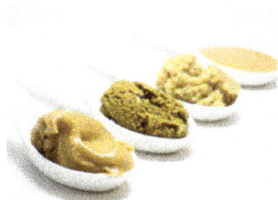

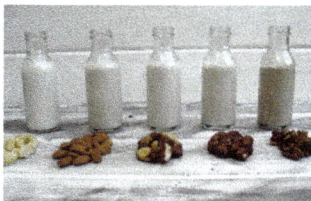

Variety of Nut Butter   Variety of Nut Milk   Cashew Nut Cheese

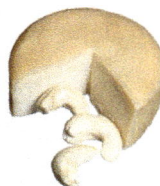

A Nutritional Powerhouse

Beyond their culinary versatility, nuts are nutritional powerhouses that provide a cornucopia of health-promoting compounds. They are a rich source of protein, fiber, healthy fats, vitamins, and minerals, making them an essential part of a balanced and nutritious diet. These nutrients work together to support various aspects of health, including:

- **Improved heart health:** Nuts are a rich source of monounsaturated and polyunsaturated fats, which help lower LDL (bad) cholesterol and raise HDL (good) cholesterol, reducing the risk of heart disease and stroke.

- **Reduced risk of chronic diseases:** Nuts contain antioxidants and anti-inflammatory compounds that help protect cells from damage and may reduce the risk of chronic diseases such as cancer, diabetes, and Alzheimer's disease.

- **Enhanced cognitive function:** Nuts are a good source of vitamin E, which is essential for brain function and may help prevent cognitive decline and memory loss.

- **Weight management:** Despite their high fat content, nuts can actually aid in weight management due to their high protein and fiber content, which promote satiety and reduce overall calorie intake.

- **Stronger bones:** Nuts contain magnesium, phosphorus, and vitamin K, all of which are important for bone health and may help reduce the risk of osteoporosis.

A Cultural Tapestry

The history of nuts is interwoven with the cultural tapestry of various civilizations around the globe. In ancient Greece and Rome, nuts were highly valued for their culinary and medicinal properties. Almonds, olives, and walnuts were particularly popular, and they were often used in religious ceremonies and offerings to deities.

Native American cultures in the southwestern United States and Mexico relied heavily on pinon pine nuts as a source of food and sustenance. These nuts were stored for use throughout the year and incorporated into traditional dishes, ceremonial practices, and medicinal remedies.

Pistachios and almonds hold a special place in Middle Eastern cuisine. In Iran, pistachios are a common ingredient in sweets, desserts, and traditional Persian ice cream. Their vibrant green color and nutty flavor add a touch of elegance and sophistication to various dishes.

Walnuts and chestnuts hold deep cultural significance in China. Walnuts are believed to promote brain health and longevity, while chestnuts are often used to treat digestive issues and are a popular winter delicacy.

In European regions, particularly Italy and France, chestnuts have been a staple food for centuries. They are often roasted and enjoyed as a snack or incorporated into savory dishes like soups and stuffing.

Nuts have also played a prominent role in African cultures for generations. Shea nuts, native to West Africa, have been valued for their medicinal properties and as a source of food and fuel. Kola nuts, also native to Africa, are considered symbols of hospitality and friendship and are often used in traditional ceremonies and rituals.

Nuts Vs Drupes: What's the Difference

Many individuals are familiar with the fact that peanuts do not fall into the category of true nuts, as they belong to the legume family. Typically, we simplify matters by labeling everything else as "tree nuts" and considering the topic settled. However, the truth is that the majority of what we commonly refer to as nuts are not true nuts at all; they are drupes.

A true nut is a fruit that consists of a hard shell and an edible seed. While in general conversation, a wide range of dried seeds are referred to as nuts, botanically speaking, there is an additional criterion: the shell must remain closed and not split open to release the seed when it reaches maturity (known as being indehiscent). Examples of "true" nuts include chestnuts and hazelnuts.

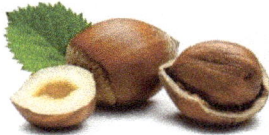

Hazelnut

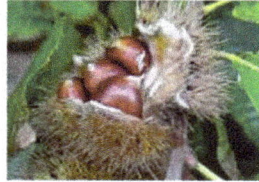

Sweet Chestnut

Nuts is botanically a specific type of fruit, but the term is also applied to many edible seeds that are not nuts in a botanical sense.

The botanical definition of a drupes fruit.

In botanical terminology, a drupe refers to a type of fruit distinguished by its outer fleshyportion, like the skin (exocarp) or flesh (mesocarp), enveloping a toughened shell (pit or stone) housing a seed. Drupes are commonly referred to as stone fruits, as each originates from a solitary carpel on a flowering plant that possesses a lone pistil.

Notably, drupes encompass various examples, including peaches, plums, and cherries. Intriguingly, walnuts, almonds, and pecans are also classified as drupes, despite their distinctive qualities.

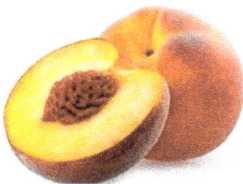

Peach

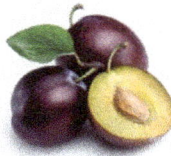

Plum

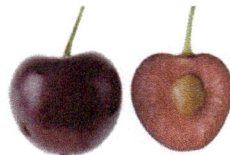

Cherries

Now, how should we categorize these diverse oily seeds that are occasionally enjoyed in their raw form and other times roasted and flavored with salt, sugar, honey, or spices such as cinnamon or chili powder? It appears that the term "culinary nuts" has become increasingly popular as a comprehensive label, which aptly captures how we commonly refer to them today.

Peanut

Although they bear the name "nut," it's important to note that peanuts are legumes. Unlike tree-grown nuts like walnuts and almonds, peanuts grow beneath the ground. Peanuts, alongside beans and peas, belong to the legume family known as Leguminosae.

Legumes are characterized by their edible seeds enclosed in pods and are recognized as a valuable source of concentrated protein within the plant kingdom.

Despite their resemblance to other legumes in terms of physical structure and nutritional benefits, peanuts are commonly incorporated into diets and cuisines in a manner like how nuts are utilized.

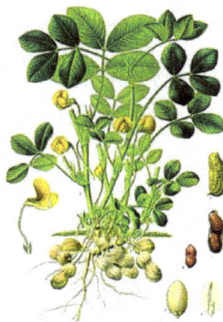

PEANUT Plant

Hopefully, the provided information has clarified any confusion that may have existed regarding nuts, drupes, and legumes.

Preparing Nuts for best Digestion

Many people enjoy nuts due to their rich reserves of healthy fats and ample protein content. These nutrient-dense snacks are not only convenient but also provide a quick and nutritious option for those with busy lifestyles.

However, many individuals lack knowledge about the best ways to enhance the digestibility of nuts. Is it essential or advantageous to consume nuts in their raw, sprouted, roasted, fried, baked, soaked, or skin-on form to maximize their nutritional value?

The answer to these queries varies depending on the individual's preferences and dietary requirements.

It is crucial to clarify the definition of "raw" when discussing nuts. In this context, "raw" refers to nuts that have been removed from their hard shells but remain uncooked, not subjected to temperatures above 46ºC.

However, this definition can cause some confusion, particularly with cashew nuts, as they are often steamed to facilitate the opening process.

- Peanuts may contain aflatoxins, a harmful fungus.

- Roasting peanuts can eliminate about half of the aflatoxins.

- Hand sorting after roasting further reduces contaminated nuts

- **Raw nuts:** Raw nuts may contain harmful bacteria and phytic acid, which can interfere with mineral absorption. Roasting, blanching, or soaking can help reduce these concerns.

- **Phytic acid:** Phytic acid is a natural compound found in nuts that can interfere with mineral absorption. Soaking nuts can help reduce phytic acid content.

- **Tannins:** Tannins are natural compounds found in nuts that give them a bitter taste. Soaking nuts can help remove tannins.

- **Goitrogens:** Goitrogens are substances that can interfere with thyroid function. Some nuts contain small amounts of goitrogens, but more research is needed to determine their effect on humans.

- **Individuals with thyroid conditions:** Individuals with thyroid conditions should exercise caution when consuming nuts, as they may exacerbate symptoms.

- **Soaking nuts:** Soaking nuts can help reduce anti-nutrient content and make them easier to digest.

Nuts are a versatile and nutritious food that can be enjoyed in many different ways. Some of the most popular ways to enjoy nuts include:

- **Soaking:** Soaking nuts in water for several hours can help to remove some of the phytic acid, which is a compound that can interfere with mineral absorption. Soaked nuts are also easier to digest than raw nuts.

- **Dehydrating:** Dehydrating nuts is a great way to preserve them for later use. Dehydrated nuts can be eaten as a snack, added to trail mix, or used in baking.

- **Activated:** Activated nuts are nuts that have been soaked and then sprouted. Sprouting nuts increases their nutritional value and makes them easier to digest.

- **Roasted:** Roasting nuts enhances their flavor and makes them more crunchy. Roasted nuts can be eaten as a snack, added to salads, or used in baking.

- **As flour:** Nut flour is a great gluten-free alternative to wheat flour. It can be used to make bread, cookies, and other baked goods.

- **As milk:** Nut milk is a dairy-free alternative to cow's milk. It is a good source of protein and calcium.

- **As oil:** Nut oil is a versatile cooking oil that can be used in a variety of dishes. It is a good source of healthy fats.

Enjoying nuts in different ways can offer various health benefits. For instance, soaked nuts can enhance nutrient absorption and ease digestion. Roasted nuts can promote a pleasant flavor and crunchiness. Moreover, nut flour can serve as a gluten-free alternative, while nut milk provides a dairy-free option. Nut oil, on the other hand, offers a versatile cooking oil with a rich source of healthy fats.

Here I now offer my humble appology to all nuts for the torture we put them through to give up their hidden secret treasures we hold a burning desires for.

Oh, the plight of the humble nut, subjected to an array of culinary trials and tribulations, all in the name of extracting your hidden treasures.

First, we force them into a milky bath, coaxing out their creamy essence.

Then, we subject them to the churning churn, transforming them into a buttery delight.

Next, we press and mold them into cheesy creations, their flavor intensifying with each squeeze.

We extract their precious oils, imbuing them with a unique fragrance and taste.

We grind them into fine flour, enabling them to weave their magic into countless culinary creations.

And finally, we infuse them into a myriad of flavors and fragrances, unlocking their aromatic potential.

Oh, the torture we put nuts through, all for the sake of our culinary pleasure. But fear not, dear nuts, for your sacrifices are not in vain.

Your hidden treasures bring joy to our palates, transforming simple meals into culinary masterpieces.

So, let us raise a toast to the humble nut, the unsung hero of our kitchens!

Conclusion

Nuts are more than just a tasty treat; they are nutritional powerhouses, culinary chameleons, and cultural treasures. Their rich history, versatility, and abundance of health benefits make them an essential part of a balanced and nutritious diet. Whether you're savoring their crunchy texture, incorporating them into your culinary creations, or enjoying their health-promoting properties, nuts are a gift from nature that should be cherished and celebrated.

Chapter Two

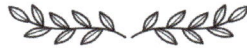

Almond - Wholesome Nut

Almonds are not only delicious but also highly regarded for their wellness and health benefits. These kernels are packed with essential nutrients that contribute to overall optimal health.

Botanically, almonds are the fruits derived from medium-sized trees belonging to the Rosaceae family and the Prunus genus.

These deciduous trees are believed to have originated in the mineral-rich mountain ranges of West Asia, where favorable conditions for their growth are abundant. Nowadays, almonds are cultivated as a significant commercial crop in various regions worldwide, including the USA.

Among the diverse array of nuts that nature has bestowed upon us, the almond stands out as a true gem. These versatile and nutritious treats, packed with essential nutrients and a delicate flavor, have captivated palates and nourished bodies for centuries. From the earliest civilizations to modern-day kitchens, almonds have been an integral part of culinary traditions and a source of health-promoting benefits.

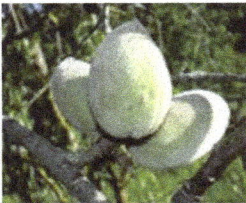

Almond Nut on Tree   Almond Nuts in Shell   Almond Out Of Shell

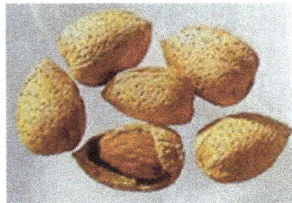

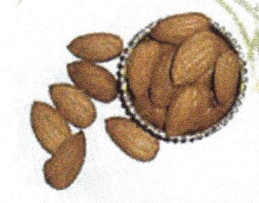

A Culinary Delight

Almonds offer a delightful culinary experience, seamlessly blending into a variety of dishes, from sweet to savory. Their crunchy texture and subtle sweetness add a touch of sophistication to salads, enhancing the flavors of fresh vegetables and leafy greens. In main courses, almonds enrich the flavors of poultry, seafood, and vegetarian dishes, providing a delightful contrast in texture. And in the realm of desserts, almonds are a star ingredient, gracing confections, pastries, and nut butters with their rich flavor and creamy texture.

A Nutritional Treasure

Beyond their culinary appeal, almonds are nutritional treasures, packed with an abundance of essential nutrients that support overall health and well-being. They are a rich source of protein, fiber, healthy fats, vitamins, and minerals, making them a valuable addition to a balanced and nutritious diet. These nutrients contribute to various health benefits, including:

- **Improved heart health:** Almonds are a rich source of monounsaturated fats, particularly oleic acid, which helps lower LDL (bad) cholesterol and raise HDL (good) cholesterol, reducing the risk of heart disease and stroke.

- **Weight management:** Despite their high fat content, almonds can actually aid in weight management due to their high protein and fiber content, which promote satiety and reduce overall calorie intake.

- **Enhanced blood sugar control:** Almonds contain fiber, magnesium, and vitamin E, all of which help regulate blood sugar levels and may reduce the risk of type 2 diabetes.

- **Strengthened bones:** Almonds are a good source of magnesium, phosphorus, and vitamin K, all of which are important for bone health and may help reduce the risk of osteoporosis.

- **Healthy skin and hair:** Almonds contain vitamin E, an antioxidant that helps protect cells from damage and may promote healthy skin and hair.

Here are some serving tips:

- Almonds can be enjoyed in various forms, whether salted, sweetened, or on their own.

- They have a delightful balance of nuttiness and pleasant sweetness. Sweetened almond milk, known as "Badam milkshake," is a popular and refreshing beverage in India and other South Asian countries.

- Almonds are highly prized and widely used in a variety of rice dishes, as well as savory and sweet preparations in the Middle East.

- Almond splits or slivers are often sprinkled over desserts, especially sundaes and other ice cream-based creations.

- They are extensively employed in confectionery, adding flavor and texture to cookies, biscuits, sweets, energy bars, and cakes. In France, almond meal is used to make an appealing cake called "frangipane."

- Blanched almond kernels are also utilized to make almond butter, providing a great alternative for individuals with peanut allergies.

A Symbol of Abundance and Prosperity

Throughout history, almonds have been associated with abundance, prosperity, and good fortune. In ancient Greece and Rome, almonds were considered a symbol of fertility and were often used in wedding ceremonies and fertility rituals. In China, almonds are considered a symbol of wealth and longevity, and they are often given as gifts during the Lunar New Year. In many cultures around the world, almonds are seen as a symbol of new beginnings and hope.

Conclusion

Almonds are more than just a delicious and nutritious food; they are culinary gems, nutritional powerhouses, and symbols of prosperity. Their versatility, abundance of health benefits, and rich cultural significance make them an essential part of a balanced diet and a source of joy to those who savor them. Whether you're sprinkling them over salads, incorporating them into main courses, or enjoying them as a simple snack, almonds are a gift from nature that should be cherished and celebrated.

Chapter Three

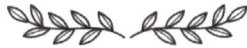

Brazil Nut - Bountiful Nut

Emerging from the lush rainforests of South America, the Brazil nut, also known as the bertholletia nut, stands as a testament to nature's bounty. These large, smooth-shelled nuts, packed with essential nutrients and a rich, buttery flavor, have captivated taste buds and nourished bodies for centuries. From the indigenous communities of the Amazon to modern-day kitchens worldwide, Brazil nuts have earned their place as a culinary treasure and a source of remarkable health benefits.

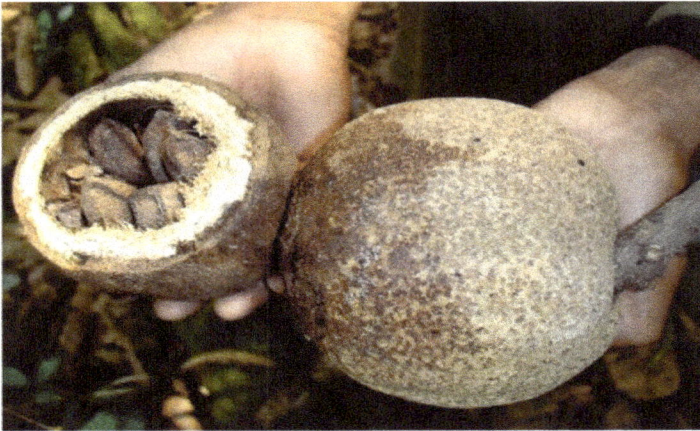

Brazil Nut in Pod

A Culinary Gem

Brazil nuts offer a unique and delightful culinary experience, gracing a variety of dishes with their rich, buttery flavor and subtly sweet undertones. Their creamy texture and delicate sweetness make them a versatile ingredient, seamlessly blending into both sweet and savory creations. In salads, they add a touch of sophistication, complementing fresh vegetables and leafy greens with their nutty richness. In main courses, they elevate the flavors of meats, poultry, and seafood, providing a luxurious contrast in texture and oil.. And in the realm of desserts, Brazil nuts are a true delight, lending their creamy texture and rich flavor to confections, pastries, and nut butters.

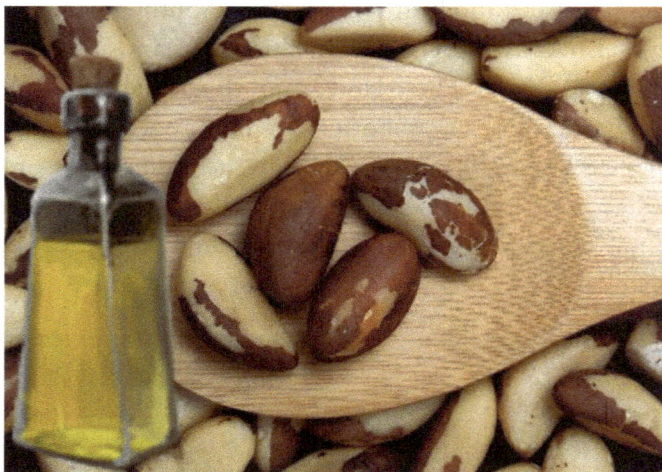

Brazil Nuts and Oil

A Nutritional Powerhouse

Beyond their culinary appeal, Brazil nuts are nutritional powerhouses, brimming with an exceptional array of essential nutrients that support overall health and well-being. They are a rich source of protein, fiber, healthy fats, vitamins, and minerals, making them an invaluable addition to a balanced and nutritious diet. These nutrients contribute to a variety of health benefits, including:

- **Superior selenium source:** Brazil nuts stand out as an extraordinary source of selenium, an essential mineral that plays a crucial role in thyroid function, immune system health, and antioxidant defense. A single Brazil nut provides nearly 100% of the daily recommended intake of selenium.

- **Enhanced heart health:** Brazil nuts are a rich source of monounsaturated and polyunsaturated fats, particularly oleic acid, which helps lower LDL (bad) cholesterol and raise HDL (good) cholesterol, reducing the risk of heart disease and stroke.

- **Improved brain function:** Brazil nuts contain magnesium, a mineral essential for cognitive function and memory, and they may help protect against age-related cognitive decline.

- **Stronger bones:** Brazil nuts are a good source of magnesium, phosphorus, and manganese, all of which are important for bone health and may help reduce the risk of osteoporosis.

- **Boosted immunity:** Brazil nuts contain vitamin E, an antioxidant that helps protect cells from damage and may enhance immune system function.

A Prized Treasure of the Amazon

Brazil nuts play a vital role in the ecology of the Amazon rainforest, serving as a food source for various wildlife species, including parrots, monkeys, and rodents. The harvesting of Brazil nuts has provided a sustainable livelihood for indigenous communities for centuries, and it continues to be an important economic activity in the region.

Conclusion

Brazil nuts are more than just a delicious and nutritious food; they are culinary gems, nutritional powerhouses, and treasures of the Amazon rainforest. Their versatility, abundance of health benefits, and significant ecological role make them an essential part of a balanced diet and a source of pride for the communities that harvest and cherish them. Whether you're savoring their rich, buttery flavor, incorporating them into your culinary creations, or appreciating their contribution to the Amazon's ecosystem, Brazil nuts are a gift from nature that should be treasured and celebrated.

Chapter Four

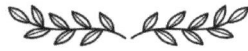

Cashew - Buttery Nut

Cashews are highly nutritious and packed with proteins and essential minerals, including copper, calcium, magnesium, iron, phosphorus, potassium, and zinc. They also contain vitamins such as C, B1 (thiamin), B2 (riboflavin), B3 (niacin), B-6, folate, E (alpha-tocopherol), and vitamin K (phylloquinone).

In addition, cashews are a source of oleic acid, providing a good quantity of monounsaturated fat and low amounts of polyunsaturated fats, with no harmful cholesterol when consumed appropriately.

These super nuts belong to the family of Anacardiaceae, which also includes mangoes and pistachios. They are originally native to the coastal areas of northeastern Brazil.

Cashews are kidney-shaped seeds and are widely cultivated in regions with tropical climates. They are grown in countries such as India, Sri Lanka, Kenya, and Tanzania. The cashew nuts stick to the bottom of their fruit, known as a cashew apple, and have various diverse uses, particularly in Brazil and some parts of Asia and Africa.

When you purchase cashews, the shells have already been removed, and they are processed for consumption. However, many people are unaware of what the original fruit looks like.

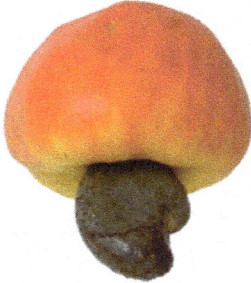

Cashew Fruit

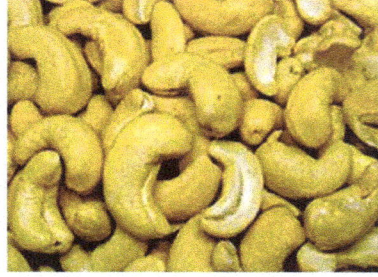

Cashew Nuts

From the lush tropical regions of the world emerges the cashew, a versatile and delectable nut that has captivated taste buds and nourished bodies for centuries. These kidney-shaped nuts, encased in a hard outer shell and boasting a rich, buttery flavor, have seamlessly integrated into culinary traditions worldwide, gracing dishes with their creamy texture and subtle sweetness. From sweet treats to savory creations, cashews are a culinary chameleon, readily adapting to a variety of flavors and cuisines.

A Culinary Delight

Cashews offer a unique and delightful culinary experience, seamlessly blending into both sweet and savory dishes with their rich, buttery flavor and subtle sweetness. Their creamy texture and versatility make them a sought-after ingredient, adding a touch of sophistication to salads, main courses, and desserts. In salads, cashews provide a delightful contrast in texture, complementing fresh vegetables and leafy greens with their nutty richness. In main courses, they enrich the flavors of poultry, seafood, and vegetarian dishes, adding a touch of indulgence to sauces and stir-fries. And in the realm of desserts, cashews are a true star, lending their creamy texture and rich flavor to confections, pastries, and nut butters.

A Nutritional Treasure Trove

Beyond their culinary appeal, cashews are nutritional treasures, packed with an abundance of essential nutrients that support overall health and well-being. They are a rich source of protein, fiber, healthy fats, vitamins, and minerals, making them an invaluable addition to a balanced and nutritious diet. These nutrients contribute to a variety of health benefits, including:

- **Improved heart health:** Cashews are a rich source of monounsaturated and polyunsaturated fats, particularly oleic acid, which helps lower LDL (bad) cholesterol and raise HDL (good) cholesterol, reducing the risk of heart disease and stroke.

- **Enhanced weight management:** Cashews contain fiber and protein, which promote satiety and help regulate appetite, making them a beneficial addition to a weight management plan.

- **Boosted cognitive function:** Cashews are a good source of copper, a mineral essential for brain function and neurotransmitter production.

- **Stronger bones:** Cashews contain magnesium, phosphorus, and manganese, all of which are important for bone health and may help reduce the risk of osteoporosis.

- **Reduced risk of chronic diseases:** Cashews contain antioxidants and anti-inflammatory compounds that help protect cells from damage and may reduce the risk of chronic diseases such as cancer, diabetes, and cardiovascular diseases.

A Versatile Ingredient in Global Cuisines

Cashews have found a home in diverse culinary traditions worldwide, seamlessly adapting to various flavors and cuisines. In Indian cuisine, cashews are a staple ingredient in curries, gravies, and sweets, adding their rich, creamy texture and subtle sweetness to traditional dishes. In Mexican cuisine, cashews are often used to make sauces and dips, lending their nutty flavor to spicy and savory creations. In Southeast Asian cuisine, cashews are a popular ingredient in stir-fries, salads, and desserts, enhancing the flavors of fresh vegetables, aromatic spices, and tropical fruits.

Conclusion

Cashews are more than just a delicious and nutritious food; they are culinary gems, nutritional powerhouses, and versatile ingredients that grace cuisines worldwide. Their adaptability, abundance of health benefits, and rich culinary heritage make them an essential part of a balanced diet and a source of inspiration for chefs and home cooks alike. Whether you're savoring their creamy texture, incorporating them into your culinary creations, or appreciating their global culinary presence, cashews are a gift from nature that should be treasured and celebrated

$\mathcal{C}hapter\ \mathcal{F}ive$

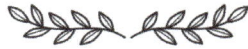

Chestnut - Wholesome Nut

Emerging from the temperate regions of the Northern Hemisphere, the chestnut, a member of the beech family, stands as a testament to nature's versatility. These round, slightly flattened nuts, encased in a prickly outer shell and boasting a sweet, starchy flavor, have played a significant role in culinary traditions and provided sustenance for centuries. From the hearths of ancient civilizations to modern-day kitchens, chestnuts have earned their place as a culinary treasure and a source of wholesome nourishment.

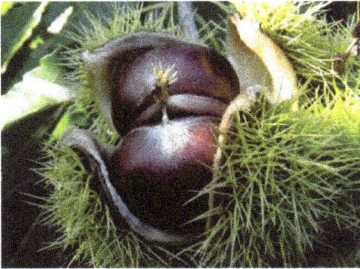

Sweet Chestnut in Pod   Horse Chestnut in Pod

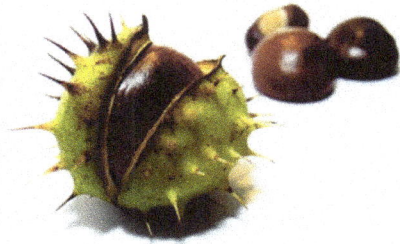

Differentiating between sweet chestnuts and toxic horse chestnuts can also be done by examining the nuts themselves. Both types are brown with a light-colored spot, but edible sweet chestnuts always have a tassel or point that can be felt by the fingers.

On the other hand, the toxic horse chestnuts are smooth and rounded without any distinct point.

Sweet chestnuts, besides being non-toxic, are also incredibly nutritious, making them an excellent choice for a healthy snack.

A Culinary Delight

Chestnuts offer a unique and delightful culinary experience, seamlessly blending into a variety of dishes with their sweet, starchy flavor and slightly nutty undertones. Their versatility makes them a sought-after ingredient, adding a touch of sophistication to both sweet and savory creations. In soups and stews, chestnuts provide a hearty texture and a rich, earthy flavor, complementing the warmth and depth of these comforting dishes. In main courses, they enrich the flavors of meats, poultry, and vegetarian dishes, lending a touch of sweetness and sophistication to traditional recipes. And in the realm of desserts, chestnuts are a true gem, gracing confections, pastries, and nut butters with their sweet, starchy appeal.

A Nutritional Powerhouse

Beyond their culinary appeal, chestnuts are nutritional powerhouses, packed with an abundance of essential nutrients that support overall health and well-being. They are a rich source of fiber, carbohydrates, vitamins, and minerals, making them an invaluable addition to a balanced and nutritious diet. These nutrients contribute to a variety of health benefits, including:

- **Improved digestive health:** Chestnuts are a rich source of fiber, which helps promote regular bowel movements, prevent constipation, and support gut health.

- **Enhanced blood sugar control:** Chestnuts contain a type of fiber called resistant starch, which helps slow down the absorption of sugar into the bloodstream, potentially benefiting individuals with diabetes.

- **Reduced risk of chronic diseases:** Chestnuts contain antioxidants and anti-inflammatory compounds that help protect cells from damage and may reduce the risk of chronic diseases such as cancer, heart disease, and type 2 diabetes.

- **Stronger bones:** Chestnuts contain potassium, magnesium, and manganese, all of which are important for bone health and may help reduce the risk of osteoporosis.

- **Improved cognitive function:** Chestnuts contain vitamin B1 (thiamine), a mineral essential for brain function and neurotransmitter production.

Chestnut Health Benefits

- Chestnuts are low in calories and fat but rich in minerals, vitamins, and phytonutrients.

- Chestnuts are primarily made of starch, providing 8.1 grams of fiber per 100 grams.

- Chestnuts are exceptionally rich in vitamin C, with 100 grams providing 72% of the Daily Recommended Intake.

- Chestnuts are a good source of folates, with 100 grams providing 15.5% of the Daily Recommended Intake.

- Chestnuts are rich in monounsaturated fatty acids, which help lower cholesterol levels.

- Chestnuts are an excellent source of minerals like potassium, iron, magnesium, and phosphorus.

- Chestnuts are a good source of B-complex vitamins niacin, pyridoxine, thiamin, and riboflavin.

- Chinese chestnuts are particularly high in vitamin A.

A Symbol of Winter and Holiday Cheer

Chestnuts have long been associated with the cozy atmosphere of winter and the festive spirit of the holiday season. Their warm, earthy flavor and hearty texture have made them a staple ingredient in traditional winter dishes, such as roasted chestnuts, chestnut stuffing, and chestnut soup. In many cultures, chestnuts are seen as a symbol of abundance, prosperity, and good fortune, often incorporated into holiday celebrations and exchanged as gifts during this special time of year.

Conclusion

Chestnuts are more than just a delicious and nutritious food; they are culinary gems, nutritional powerhouses, and symbols of winter and holiday cheer. Their versatility, abundance of health benefits, and rich cultural significance make them an essential part of a balanced diet and a source of inspiration for chefs and home cooks alike. Whether you're savoring their warm, earthy flavor, incorporating them into your holiday feasts, or appreciating their cultural symbolism, chestnuts are a gift from nature that should be treasured and celebrated.

Chapter Six

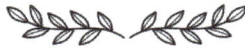

Horse Chestnut – Revitalizing Nut

Native to the Balkan Peninsula but widely distributed throughout the Northern Hemisphere, the horse chestnut, scientifically known as Aesculus hippocastanum, is a majestic tree with distinctive palmate leaves and large, brown conkers. While the conkers are not edible for humans, the seeds within them hold potential therapeutic properties.

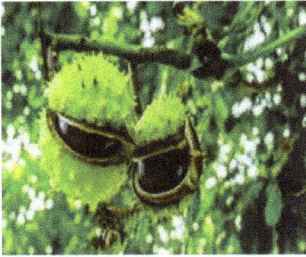

Horse Chestnut In Pod on Tree

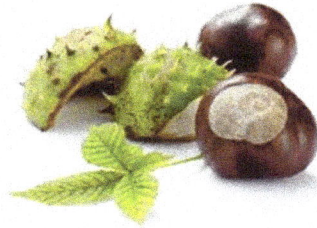

Horse Chestnut Out of Pod

Traditional Uses and Scientific Evidence

For centuries, various parts of the horse chestnut tree, including seeds, leaves, bark, and flowers, have been used in folk medicine to address various ailments. While some of these traditional uses lack scientific backing, the seeds have garnered attention for their potential benefits in managing chronic venous insufficiency (CVI).

CVI is a condition characterized by impaired blood flow in the veins, often resulting in symptoms such as varicose veins, swelling, pain, and fatigue. Horse chestnut seed extract, prepared to remove the toxic substance esculin, has been shown to exhibit similar effects to compression stockings, helping to contract veins and reduce fluid buildup.

Mechanism of Action

The therapeutic properties of horse chestnut seed extract are attributed to its active compounds, primarily aescin. Aescin is believed to exert various actions, including:

- Reducing inflammation
- Enhancing blood vessel tone
- Improving blood flow
- Promoting fluid drainage
- Strengthening capillary walls

Clinical Studies and Safety Considerations

Research has provided promising evidence for the effectiveness of horse chestnut seed extract in managing CVI symptoms. A study published in the Lancet compared horse chestnut seed extract to compression stockings and found both treatments equally effective in improving symptoms.

While horse chestnut seed extract is generally considered safe for short-term use under proper guidance, it is crucial to note that raw consumption of horse chestnut seeds or unprocessed extracts can be toxic due to the presence of esculin. Pregnant or breastfeeding women, individuals with kidney or liver disorders, and those taking blood thinners should consult their healthcare provider before using horse chestnut extract.

Topical Applications and Alternative Therapies

While the use of horse chestnut seed extract may hold some promise for CVI, topical applications of horse chestnut leaf or bark extracts have shown some benefits for various skin conditions, such as eczema, ulcers, and sprains.

Alternative therapies that may complement the use of horse chestnut extract for CVI include:

- Regular exercise
- Weight management
- Compression stockings
- Elevated legs
- Dietary modifications

Conclusion

Horse chestnut, particularly its seed extract, has emerged as a promising natural remedy for chronic venous insufficiency. Its ability to improve blood flow, reduce inflammation, and strengthen capillary walls makes it a valuable tool in managing CVI symptoms. However, it is essential to consult with a healthcare provider before using horse chestnut extract, as it may interact with certain medications or health conditions.

Chapter Seven

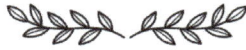

Coconut – Tropical Re-freshness

Native to tropical and subtropical regions worldwide, the coconut palm (Cocos nucifera) is a symbol of tropical paradise and a versatile source of nourishment. Its distinctive fruit, the coconut, is a botanical wonder, categorized as a drupe rather than a nut. Celebrated for its remarkable versatility and rich nutritional profile, the coconut has played a vital role in human civilization for centuries.

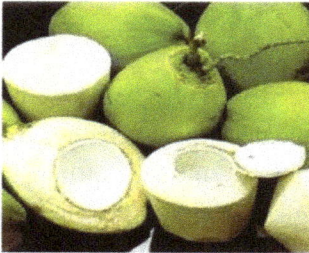

Young Coconut with jelly and water   Mature Coconut

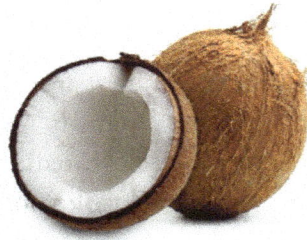

A Culinary Delight and a Nutritional Powerhouse

Coconuts are an integral part of many people's daily diets, offering a unique blend of flavors and textures. When immature, they are known as tender-nuts or jelly-nuts and can be harvested for their refreshing, slightly sweet water. As they mature, they retain some water and can be used as seednuts or processed to extract oil from the kernel.

Beyond its culinary appeal, the coconut stands out as a nutritional powerhouse, providing an abundance of essential nutrients that support overall health and well-being. It is a rich source of fiber, vitamins, and minerals, including:

- Dietary fiber: Coconut is an excellent source of dietary fiber, which helps promote digestive health, regulate blood sugar levels, and contribute to weight management.

- Vitamins: Coconuts are a good source of vitamins C, E, and B-complex vitamins, which play crucial roles in various bodily functions, including immune system support, antioxidant protection, and energy production.

- Minerals: Coconuts are rich in minerals such as iron, magnesium, potassium, and manganese, which are essential for blood health, muscle and nerve function, bone health, and various metabolic processes.

A Versatile Fruit with Diverse Applications

The versatility of the coconut extends far beyond its culinary and nutritional value. Its various parts have been utilized for a wide range of purposes throughout history. The fibrous husk, or mesocarp, is often used for making ropes, mats, and other household items. The shell, or endocarp, can be crafted into bowls, utensils, and musical instruments.

Coconut oil, extracted from the kernel, has gained immense popularity in recent years due to its numerous health benefits. It is a rich source of healthy fats, particularly medium-chain triglycerides (MCTs), which have been shown to improve cognitive function, boost metabolism, and promote weight loss.

A Cultural Icon and a Symbol of Sustainability

The coconut holds deep cultural significance in many tropical societies, where it is considered a symbol of abundance, prosperity, and hospitality. Coconut palms are often revered as sacred trees, and their various parts are used in traditional medicine, ceremonies, and artistic expressions.

In addition to its cultural significance, the coconut tree plays a vital role in sustainable agriculture and environmental protection. Its deep root system helps prevent soil erosion, and its leaves provide shade and habitat for various wildlife species. Coconut trees are also a valuable source of renewable energy, as their fibrous husks can be used to produce biofuels.

Coconut – A Treasure Trove of Health

The coconut, a versatile and nutritious fruit native to tropical and subtropical regions, has long been revered for its culinary, cultural, and medicinal significance. Its unique composition, rich in medium-chain triglycerides (MCTs), sets it apart from other sources of fats and oils, offering a range of health benefits.

Nutritional Profile and Therapeutic Properties

Coconuts are a rich source of essential nutrients, including fiber, vitamins, and minerals. They are particularly well-known for their high MCT content, which provides a quick source of energy and supports various bodily functions.

MCTs have been shown to:

- Enhance cognitive function and memory

- Boost metabolism and promote weight loss

- Support immune system function

- Exhibit antibacterial and antiviral properties

Traditional medicine has long recognized the therapeutic potential of coconuts and their derived products. Coconut oil, for instance, has been used to treat a wide range of ailments, including skin infections, digestive issues, and respiratory problems.

Modern Scientific Insights and Health Implications

Recent scientific studies have provided further evidence supporting the health benefits of coconuts. Research suggests that:

- Coconut consumption may protect against heart disease and stroke by reducing LDL cholesterol levels.

- MCTs from coconuts may offer an alternative energy source for the brain, potentially benefiting individuals with neurological disorders.

- Coconut water, with its abundance of electrolytes, can help prevent and treat dehydration caused by various conditions.

Culinary Versatility and Practical Applications

Coconuts are remarkably versatile, offering a variety of culinary and practical applications. Their tender meat can be enjoyed raw, cooked, or preserved, adding a subtle sweetness and nutty flavor to various dishes. Coconut water, a refreshing beverage, provides natural hydration and replenishes essential electrolytes.

Beyond its culinary uses, the coconut tree provides a range of practical benefits:

- Its fibrous husk is used for making ropes, mats, and other household items.

- The shell is crafted into bowls, utensils, and musical instruments.

- Coconut oil is a valuable source of renewable energy, as it can be converted into biofuels.

Coconut - A Nutritional Powerhouse and Culinary Delight

The coconut, a versatile and nutritious fruit native to tropical and subtropical regions, has long been revered for its culinary, cultural, and medicinal significance. Its unique composition, rich in medium-chain triglycerides (MCTs), sets it apart from other sources of fats and oils, offering a range of health benefits and culinary applications.

A Nutrient-Dense Fruit with Diverse Culinary Uses

Coconuts are a rich source of essential nutrients, including fiber, vitamins, and minerals. They are particularly well-known for their high MCT content, which provides a quick source of energy and supports various bodily functions.

Beyond its nutritional value, the coconut is remarkably versatile in the kitchen. Its tender meat can be enjoyed raw, cooked, or preserved, adding a subtle sweetness and nutty flavor to various dishes. Coconut water, a refreshing beverage, provides natural hydration and replenishes essential electrolytes.

Coconut Milk: A Lactose-Free Alternative and Culinary Staple

Coconut milk, derived from the grated flesh of the coconut and soaked in hot water, serves as a lactose-free alternative to cow's milk and a versatile ingredient in various cuisines. Its rich and creamy texture enhances curries, soups, smoothies, and desserts.

Coconut Oil: A Culinary Staple with Health-Promoting Properties

Coconut oil, extracted from the dried coconut meat, has gained immense popularity in recent years due to its numerous health benefits and wide range of culinary applications. Its high smoke point makes it suitable for high-heat cooking methods, and its unique fatty acid composition offers various health advantages.

MCTs: The Key to Coconut Oil's Unique Benefits

MCTs, the predominant fatty acids in coconut oil, are metabolized differently than long-chain fatty acids (LCFAs) found in most other oils. They are readily absorbed by the liver and converted into energy, providing a quick and sustained source of fuel.

Health Benefits of Coconut Oil

Research has uncovered several health benefits associated with coconut oil, including:

- **Improved cognitive function:** MCTs may enhance cognitive function and memory.

- **Boosted metabolism:** MCTs may help boost metabolism and promote weight loss.

- **Strengthened immune system:** Lauric acid, a prominent MCT in coconut oil, may enhance immune function by fighting harmful microorganisms.

- **Antimicrobial and antifungal properties:** Coconut oil exhibits antimicrobial and antifungal properties, potentially aiding in wound healing and infection prevention.

Coconut Oil: A Culinary and Therapeutic Treasure

Coconut oil's versatility extends beyond its nutritional value and health benefits. Its unique properties make it a valuable ingredient in various cosmetic and medicinal applications, including skin care, hair care, and massage therapy.

Conclusion

The coconut, a fruit with a rich history and diverse applications, continues to be a source of nourishment, cultural significance, and scientific intrigue. Its unique composition, offering both culinary delights and a range of health benefits, makes it a truly remarkable fruit that enriches lives around the world.

African Palm Nut (Elaeis guineensis)

Palm nuts are an important food source in many tropical regions around the world, providing nourishment and cultural significance to various communities. Among the diverse palm nut varieties, the African oil palm nut (Elaeis guineensis) holds a prominent position. Native to West and Southwest Africa, specifically the area between Angola and The Gambia, this species is the primary source of palm oil, a versatile oil used in various industries.

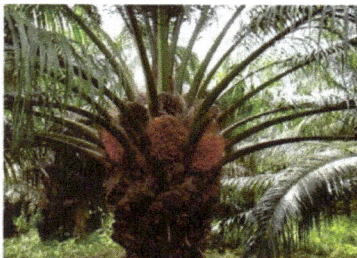

African Palm Nut on Tree

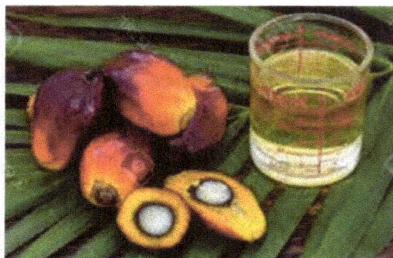

Palm Nut open with oil Produced

Characteristics and Uses of African Palm Nut

African palm nuts are typically high in fat and protein, offering a rich source of energy and essential nutrients. They contain a variety of vitamins and minerals, making them a valuable addition to traditional diets. Palm nuts are often incorporated into traditional dishes such as curries and stews, adding a unique flavor and texture. Additionally, they can be roasted and enjoyed as a nutritious snack.

Beyond their culinary applications, palm nuts have gained significance in various industries. Palm oil, extracted from the African oil palm nut, is widely used in the food and cosmetics industries. Its versatility and affordability have made it a popular ingredient in cooking oils, margarine, and various processed foods. Additionally, palm oil finds application in the production of soaps, detergents, and cosmetics.

Environmental Considerations and Sustainable Practices

The production of palm oil, particularly in Southeast Asia, has raised concerns about deforestation and habitat destruction. The expansion of palm oil plantations has led to the clearing of vast areas of tropical forests, impacting biodiversity and disrupting ecosystems. These concerns have sparked environmental and social movements advocating for sustainable palm oil production practices.

Sustainable palm oil production aims to minimize the environmental and social impacts of the industry. This approach involves practices such as:

- **Efficient land use:** Optimizing land utilization to maximize palm oil production while minimizing deforestation.

- **Wildlife conservation:** Implementing measures to protect endangered species and conserve natural habitats within palm oil plantations.

- **Social responsibility:** Ensuring fair labor practices, respecting indigenous rights, and improving the livelihoods of communities affected by palm oil production.

The adoption of sustainable practices is crucial for mitigating the negative impacts of palm oil production and ensuring the long-term sustainability of the industry. By balancing economic growth with environmental and social considerations, sustainable palm oil

Halsey Cruickshank

production can contribute to a more harmonious relationship between human activities and the natural world.

Chapter Eight

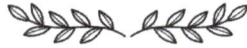

Hazelnuts – Irresistible Nut

Hazelnuts, the edible nuts derived from various species of hazel trees belonging to the genus Corylus, have long been prized for their nutritional value, culinary versatility, and cultural significance. Their unique composition, rich in essential nutrients and beneficial compounds, offers a range of health benefits and culinary applications.

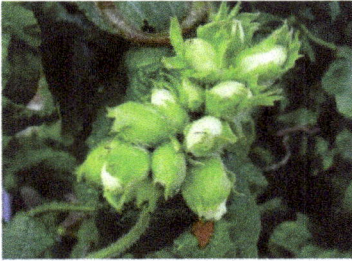

Hazel nut developing on tree

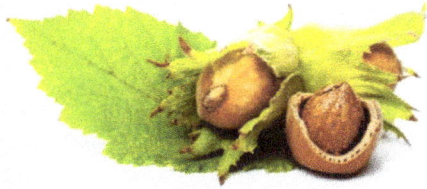

Hazel nut in shell

Botanical Characteristics and Cultivation

Hazelnuts are typically harvested from the Corylus avellana species, commonly known as the European filbert or cobnut. These nuts are characterized by their round to oval shape, enclosed within a fibrous husk that naturally falls off when ripe. The edible kernel within the shell is typically light brown in color and possesses a slightly sweet, nutty flavor.

Hazelnut trees thrive in temperate climates, preferring well-drained soils and ample sunlight. They are primarily cultivated in regions with mild winters and warm summers, with Turkey, Italy, Georgia, and Azerbaijan being among the top hazelnut-producing countries globally.

Nutritional Profile and Health Benefits

Hazelnuts are a rich source of essential nutrients, including:

- **Monounsaturated fats:** Hazelnuts are notably high in monounsaturated fatty acids, particularly oleic acid, which is associated with improved heart health and reduced risk of cardiovascular diseases.

- **Vitamin E:** Hazelnuts are an excellent source of vitamin E, a potent antioxidant that protects cells from damage and may contribute to cancer prevention.

- **Folate:** Hazelnuts are particularly rich in folate, a B vitamin essential for DNA synthesis and crucial for preventing neural tube defects in newborns.

- **Dietary fiber:** Hazelnuts are a good source of dietary fiber, which promotes digestive health, regulates blood sugar levels, and contributes to a feeling of fullness.

- **Minerals:** Hazelnuts are a rich source of minerals, including manganese, copper, magnesium, potassium, and calcium, all of which play essential roles in various bodily functions.

Culinary Versatility and Applications

Hazelnuts are remarkably versatile culinary ingredients, enjoyed in various forms and incorporated into a wide range of dishes. They can be consumed raw, roasted, or ground into a paste, adding a nutty flavor and crunchy texture to various culinary creations.

- **Confectionery:** Hazelnuts are widely used in confectionery, often paired with chocolate in delicacies like pralines, truffles, and Nutella.

- **Baking:** Hazelnuts are a popular ingredient in baking, adding a delightful crunch and nutty flavor to cookies, cakes, breads, and pastries.

- **Sauces and dressings:** Hazelnut oil, extracted from the nuts, is a valuable ingredient in sauces and dressings, imparting a rich, nutty flavor that complements various dishes.

- **Dairy alternatives:** Hazelnut milk and hazelnut butter offer dairy-free alternatives for those with lactose intolerance or nut allergies.

Potential Health Concerns and Considerations

While hazelnuts offer a wealth of health benefits, it is essential to consume them in moderation as part of a balanced diet. Their high fat content, particularly monounsaturated fats, can contribute to increased calorie intake. Additionally, individuals with hazelnut allergies should strictly avoid consuming hazelnuts or products containing them.

Conclusion

Hazelnuts, with their unique nutritional profile, culinary versatility, and rich cultural significance, stand as a testament to nature's bounty. Their combination of essential nutrients, health-promoting compounds, and delightful flavor makes them a valuable addition to a balanced diet and a culinary delight that continues to enrich cuisines worldwide.

Chapter Nine

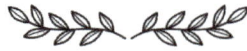

Macadamia – Luxurious Nut

M acadamia nuts, native to the rainforests of northeastern Australia, have captivated the world with their unique flavor and remarkable nutritional profile. These buttery, smooth-textured nuts, cultivated in various tropical and subtropical regions worldwide, hold a prominent position among edible nuts, offering a delectable treat and a rich source of essential nutrients.

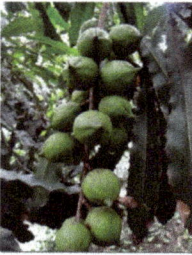

Macadamia nut on tree

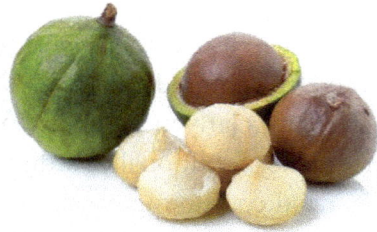

Macadamia Nuts in and out of Pod

Botanical Characteristics and Cultivation

Macadamia trees, belonging to the Proteaceae family, are distinguished by their evergreen foliage and creamy-white flowers that bloom in elongated racemes. The nuts, enclosed in a tough outer shell, typically ripen around the seventh year of plantation.

Nutritional Profile and Health Benefits

Macadamia nuts are a treasure trove of nutrients, including:

- **Monounsaturated fats:** Rich in oleic acid and palmitoleic acids, macadamia nuts contribute to improved heart health by reducing LDL cholesterol levels and promoting arterial health.

- **Antioxidants:** Macadamia nuts contain vitamin A, vitamin E, and flavonoids, which act as antioxidants, protecting cells from damage caused by free radicals. These antioxidants are associated with a reduced risk of chronic diseases, including certain types of cancer.

- **Fiber:** With a significant amount of soluble and insoluble fiber, macadamia nuts promote digestive health, regulate blood sugar levels, and aid in weight management.

- **Other essential nutrients:** Macadamia nuts are a good source of protein, minerals such as magnesium, manganese, calcium, and iron, and B vitamins, all of which play vital roles in various bodily functions.

Culinary Applications and Versatility

Macadamia nuts are culinary delights, adding a rich, buttery flavor and a satisfying crunch to various dishes. They can be:

- **Eaten raw:** Enjoyed as a snack or incorporated into trail mixes and granola bars.

- **Roasted and salted:** Enhance the flavor of salads, desserts, and savory dishes.

- **Ground into paste:** Used as a spread or incorporated into baked goods, adding a nutty flavor and moist texture.

- **Macadamia oil:** Derived from the nuts, macadamia oil possesses a delicate flavor and high smoke point, making it suitable for cooking and dressing various dishes.

Considerations and Potential Concerns

While macadamia nuts offer an array of health benefits, it is essential to consume them in moderation as part of a balanced diet. Their high fat content, particularly monounsaturated fats, can contribute to increased calorie intake. Additionally, individuals with nut allergies should strictly avoid consuming macadamia nuts or products containing them.

Macadamia Nut Oil: A Culinary Delight with Health-Promoting Properties

Macadamia nut oil, derived from the buttery, smooth-textured macadamia nuts, has gained recognition for its unique flavor, culinary versatility, and remarkable health benefits. Its well-balanced ratio of omega-3 and omega-6 fatty acids, along with its abundance of antioxidants and phytochemicals, makes it a valuable addition to a balanced diet.

Health Benefits: A Symphony of Wellness

The incorporation of macadamia nut oil into your diet may offers a range of health benefits:

- **Heart Health:** The favorable fatty acid profile of macadamia nut oil helps lower LDL cholesterol, reducing the risk of cardiovascular diseases.

- **Cancer Prevention:** Antioxidants and phytochemicals in macadamia nut oil protect cells from damage, potentially reducing the risk of certain types of cancer.

- **Skin Health:** Macadamia nut oil's high antioxidant content and resemblance to sebum make it an excellent moisturizer for the skin, helping to prevent dryness and delay the signs of aging.

- **Hair Health:** Macadamia nut oil nourishes and strengthens hair follicles, promoting healthy hair growth and reducing hair loss.

- **Immune System Support:** Macadamia nut oil's antioxidants and phytochemicals contribute to a robust immune system, helping the body fight off infections and illnesses.

Conclusion

Macadamia nuts, with their unique combination of flavor, nutritional value, and culinary versatility, stand as a testament to nature's bounty. Their ability to provide essential nutrients, promote heart health, and enhance the taste of various dishes makes them a valuable addition to a balanced diet and a culinary delight enjoyed worldwide.

Chapter Ten

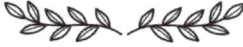

Pecan – Decadent Nut

Pecans, the nuts of the pecan tree (Carya illinoinensis), are a prized culinary treasure and a rich source of essential nutrients. Native to central and southern regions of the United States, pecans have been cultivated worldwide for their unique flavor, nutritional value, and culinary versatility.

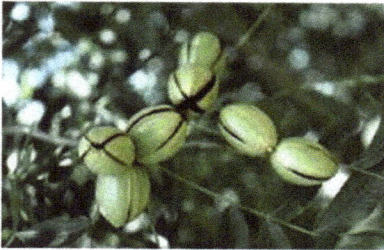

Pecan Fruit

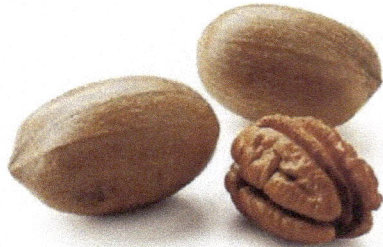

Pecan in & out of shell

A Culinary Delight with a Rich History

Pecans, named after an Algonquian word meaning "a nut that requires a stone to crack," have been savored by Native Americans for centuries. Their buttery, sweet taste and high-fat content make them a versatile ingredient in a variety of dishes, from savory snacks to decadent desserts.

Nutritional Powerhouse: A Symphony of Health Benefits

Pecans are not just a delightful treat; they are packed with essential nutrients that contribute to overall health. Their high content of monounsaturated fats, particularly oleic acid, has been linked to improved heart health by reducing LDL cholesterol levels and promoting arterial health.

Pecans are also a rich source of antioxidants and phytochemicals, including vitamin E, beta-carotene, lutein, zeaxanthin, and ellagic acid. These compounds help protect cells from damage caused by free radicals, potentially reducing the risk of chronic diseases such as cancer and heart disease.

Culinary Versatility:

- Pecans can be cooked into a variety of dishes, including pies, fudge, baklava, muffins, and pecan caramel puddles.
- They can also be used to make pecan nut butter and are a popular topping for sundaes and bourbon ice creams.

Health Benefits:

- Pecans are a good source of monounsaturated fats, fiber, and antioxidants.
- They can help to improve heart health by reducing LDL cholesterol levels and promoting arterial health.
- They are also a rich source of vitamin E, beta-carotene, lutein, zeaxanthin, and ellagic acid, which help to protect cells from damage caused by free radicals. • Cooking Oil:
- Pecan oil is a versatile cooking oil with a neutral flavor that can be used for high-temperature cooking and deep frying.
- It is rich in monounsaturated fats and has a high smoke point of 470 degrees Fahrenheit. • Selection and Storage:
- Pecan nuts are available shelled, unshelled, salted, and sweetened.

- They can be stored in a cool, dry place for several months.

- Shelled pecans should be kept in an airtight container in the refrigerator to prevent them from becoming rancid.

Conclusion: A Nutty Gem with Culinary and Health Benefits

Pecans, with their unique flavor profile, remarkable nutritional value, and culinary versatility, stand as a testament to nature's bounty. Their ability to enhance heart health, promote skin and hair health, and provide essential nutrients makes them a valuable addition to a balanced diet and a culinary delight enjoyed worldwide. Whether you're seeking a healthy cooking oil or a flavor enhancer for your culinary creations, pecans offer a symphony of taste and health benefits.

Chapter Eleven

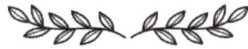

Penuts – Nutrilicious Nut

Peanuts, also known as groundnuts (Arachis hypogaea), are a crop of global importance, widely grown in tropical and subtropical regions. They hold significance for both small-scale and large-scale commercial producers. Classified as both a grain legume and an oil crop due to their high oil content, peanuts hold a unique position in the agricultural world.

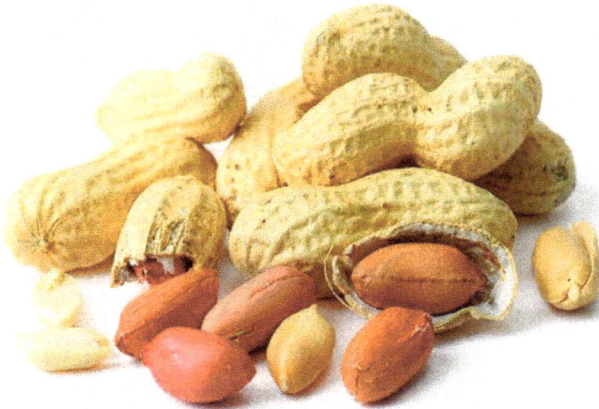

Peanuts (courtesy the harvest club.org)

Cultivar Groups: A Diverse Array of Peanuts

Several peanut cultivars are grown worldwide, each with unique characteristics and adaptations. Four major cultivar groups dominate global peanut production:

1. **Spanish Group:** Known for their small kernels and reddish-brown skin, Spanish peanuts are primarily used in candies, peanut butter, and salted nuts. They have a higher oil content compared to other types and are mainly grown in New Mexico, Oklahoma, and Texas in the U.S.

2. **Runner Group:** This group encompasses a wide range of peanut varieties, including the popular "Florunner." Runners are known for their large kernels, attractive appearance, good flavor, and superior roasting qualities. They are widely grown in Georgia, Alabama, Florida, Texas, and Oklahoma, accounting for approximately 80% of total U.S. peanut production.

3. **Virginia Group:** Virginia peanuts boast the largest kernels among cultivars, making them ideal for processing, salting, confectionery uses, and in-shell roasting. They are primarily cultivated in southeastern Virginia, northeastern North Carolina, and West Texas, accounting for about 15% of total U.S. peanut production.

4. **Valencia Group:** Valencia peanuts typically have three or more small kernels per pod. They are known for their sweetness and are often roasted and sold in the shell, making them excellent for fresh use as boiled peanuts. Valencia peanuts are not as widely cultivated in the U.S., accounting for less than 1% of total production. They are mainly grown in New Mexico..

Peanut Production and Trade

- The world produced 29 million metric tons of peanuts per year.
- China produces about 37% of world peanut production.
- The major peanut exporters are India, Argentina, the United States, China, and Malawi.

- The major peanut importers are the Netherlands, Indonesia, Mexico, Germany, and Russia.
- Canada, Mexico, Europe, and Japan account for over 80% of U.S. exports.

Health Benefits of Peanuts:

Peanuts offer a wealth of health benefits due to their rich nutrient content:

1. Protein Powerhouse: Peanuts are a plant-based protein source, providing about 7.6 grams of protein per handful. They are also a good source of arginine, an amino acid that plays a role in wound healing, immune function, and blood vessel dilation.

2. Heart-Healthy Fats: Peanuts contain monounsaturated fatty acids, particularly oleic acid, which helps lower LDL (bad) cholesterol and raise HDL (good) cholesterol levels. Studies suggest that incorporating peanuts into a healthy diet can reduce the risk of heart disease by up to 50%.

3. Essential Vitamins and Minerals: Peanuts are packed with essential vitamins and minerals, including vitamin E, niacin, thiamin, pantothenic acid, vitamin B6, folate, copper, manganese, potassium, calcium, iron, magnesium, zinc, phosphorus, and selenium.

4. Potential Cancer-Protective Effects: Research indicates that peanuts' high concentration of polyphenolic antioxidants, particularly p-coumaric acid and resveratrol, may help reduce the risk of stomach cancer and other degenerative diseases.

5. Enhanced Antioxidant Bioavailability: Roasting or boiling peanuts can increase their antioxidant bioavailability, making it easier for the body to absorb these beneficial compounds.

The following text is a comprehensive overview of peanuts, including their cultivation, nutritional benefits, culinary applications, and potential health risks. Here's a summary of the key points:

- **Types of Peanuts:** Peanuts belong to the Fabaceae family and are classified into four main cultivar groups: Spanish, Runner, Virginia, and Valencia. Each group has unique characteristics and is suited for different culinary purposes.

- **Health Benefits of Peanuts:** Peanuts offer a wealth of health benefits due to their rich nutrient content. They are a good source of protein, healthy fats, essential vitamins and minerals, and polyphenolic antioxidants.

- **Peanut Flour Uses:** Peanut flour is a versatile ingredient used in baking, marinades, sauces, and as a gluten-free alternative to wheat flour.

- **Peanut Selection and Storage:** Choose peanuts with compact, off-white color, a healthy-looking shell, and a uniform size. Store peanuts in a cool, dry place to prevent spoilage.

- **Peanut Allergy and Hypersensitivity:** Some individuals may experience severe allergic reactions to peanuts, manifesting as symptoms like vomiting, stomach pain, swelling, and breathing difficulties. Avoid peanuts if you suspect an allergy.

- **Peanut Oil Health Benefits:** Peanut oil is a good source of vitamin E and monounsaturated fats, which may help lower cholesterol levels and reduce the risk of heart disease.

- **Peanut Oil Safety:** Peanut oil is not safe for individuals with peanut allergies. It is crucial to check food labels and notify servers when dining out if you have a peanut allergy.

- **Peanut Allergy Prevention:** Guidelines suggest that early introduction of peanut-containing foods to infants may help prevent the development of peanut allergies.

- **Peanut Nutritional Information:** One ounce of peanuts provides approximately 161 calories, 7 grams of protein, 14 grams of fat (mostly unsaturated), and essential vitamins and minerals.

Conclusion: A Nut with Global Significance

Peanuts, with their versatility, nutritional value, and adaptability to diverse growing conditions, have earned a significant place in global agriculture. Their ability to enhance culinary creations, provide essential nutrients, and serve as a raw material for various products ensures their continued importance in the world of food and agriculture. Whether savored in their natural form, transformed into peanut butter, or incorporated into culinary delights, peanuts remain a beloved nut with global significance.

Chapter Twelve

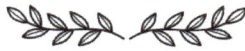

Pine Nut – Elevator Nut

ine nuts, botanically classified as Pinus pinea, are edible seeds produced by pine trees. They are also known as pignolia, cedar nuts, or piñones. Pine nuts have been a prized culinary ingredient for centuries, valued for their delicate flavor, crunchy texture, and rich nutrient content.

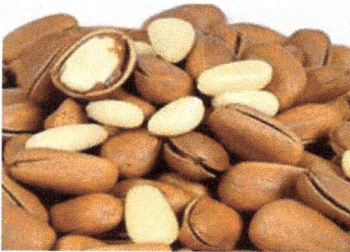

Pine Nuts in and out of shell

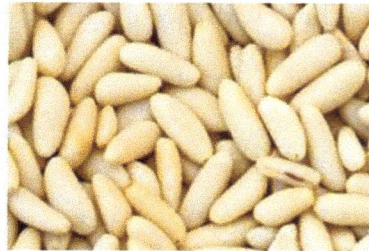

Pine nut out of shell

Cultivation and Varieties:

Pine nuts are derived from various pine tree species, with Pinus pinea being the most commercially cultivated variety. These trees are native to the Mediterranean region, particularly in Italy, Spain, Portugal, and Turkey. Pine trees typically take around 20-30 years to mature and produce cones containing the edible seeds.

Nutritional Profile:

Pine nuts are a nutrient-dense food, offering a wealth of health benefits. They are an excellent source of protein, providing approximately 3 grams per ounce. Pine nuts also contain healthy fats, primarily monounsaturated and polyunsaturated fatty acids, which contribute to heart health and may lower cholesterol levels. Additionally, they are rich in dietary fiber, essential vitamins and minerals, including vitamin E, magnesium, manganese, potassium, and iron.

Culinary Applications:

Pine nuts are highly versatile ingredients, adding a unique flavor and texture to various culinary creations. They are commonly used in pesto, a classic Italian sauce, and are often incorporated into salads, pasta dishes, and risottos. Pine nuts also enhance the flavor of baked goods, such as cookies, cakes, and breads. Their mild nutty flavor pairs well with various cheeses, dried fruits, and herbs.

Health Benefits:

Beyond their culinary value, pine nuts offer a range of health benefits:

- **Heart Health:** The monounsaturated and polyunsaturated fats in pine nuts may help lower LDL (bad) cholesterol and raise HDL (good) cholesterol levels, reducing the risk of heart disease.

- **Antioxidant Protection:** Pine nuts are rich in vitamin E, a potent antioxidant that helps protect cells from damage caused by free radicals.

- **Weight Management:** Pine nuts are a good source of protein and fiber, which can promote satiety and aid in weight management.

- **Mineral Richness:** Pine nuts provide essential minerals like magnesium, manganese, potassium, and iron, which play crucial roles in various bodily functions.

Selection and Storage:

When selecting pine nuts, choose those with a uniform size, creamy white color, and a pleasant nutty aroma. Avoid nuts with blemishes, discoloration, or a rancid smell. Store pine nuts in an airtight container in a cool, dark place to preserve their freshness and prevent spoilage.

Potential Allergic Reactions:

While pine nuts are generally safe for consumption, some individuals may experience allergic reactions. Symptoms of pine nut allergy can range from mild, such as itching or tingling, to severe, including swelling, difficulty breathing, and anaphylaxis. If you suspect a pine nut allergy, consult a healthcare professional for proper diagnosis and management.

Conclusion:

Pine nuts are a culinary delight and a nutritional powerhouse, offering a rich flavor, crunchy texture, and a variety of health benefits. Their versatility in various culinary creations and their positive impact on health make pine nuts a valuable addition to a balanced diet.

Chapter Thirteen

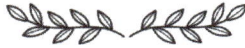

Pistachio - Vibrant Nut

The pistachio is a small tree originating from Central Asia and the Middle East. Its seeds, or nuts, are widely consumed as food and have been revered for their nutritional value since ancient times. This chapter explores the cultivation, nutritional profile, health benefits, culinary applications, and selection and storage of pistachios.

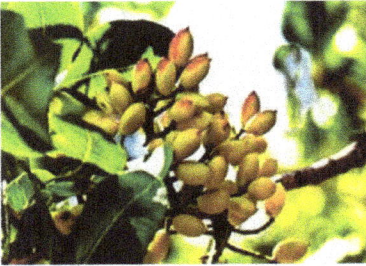

Pistacia vera (Kerman cultivar) fruits ripening

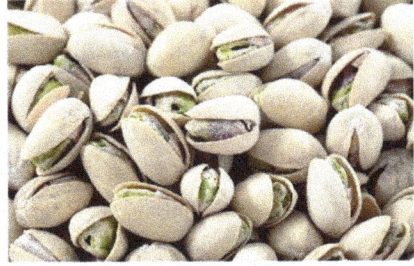

Open Pistachio nuts

Nutritional Profile

Pistachios are a rich source of essential nutrients, including:

- **Protein:** Pistachios provide approximately 6 grams of protein per ounce, contributing to satiety and muscle development.

- **Healthy Fats:** Pistachios contain predominantly monounsaturated and polyunsaturated fats, which are beneficial for heart health and may lower LDL (bad) cholesterol levels.

- **Dietary Fiber:** Pistachios offer around 3 grams of dietary fiber per ounce, promoting digestive health and aiding in weight management.

- **Vitamins and Minerals:** Pistachios are an excellent source of vitamins E, B6, potassium, copper, manganese, and magnesium.

Health Benefits

Regular consumption of pistachios is associated with a range of health benefits, including:

- **Heart Health:** Pistachios may help lower LDL (bad) cholesterol and raise HDL (good) cholesterol, reducing the risk of heart disease.

- **Weight Management:** Pistachios' high protein, fiber, and healthy fat content promote satiety and may aid in weight management.

- **Eye Health:** Pistachios contain lutein and zeaxanthin, antioxidants that may help reduce the risk of age-related macular degeneration (AMD).

- **Skin Health:** Pistachios contain saturated fats that help keep the skin hydrated and may alleviate dryness.

- **Digestive Health:** Pistachios' dietary fiber promotes smooth digestion and regularity.

- **Sexual Vitality:** Research suggests that pistachios may improve erectile function in men.

- **Antioxidant Protection:** Pistachios contain antioxidants that help protect cells from damage caused by free radicals.

- **Potential Diabetes Defense:** Pistachios' antioxidants may help reduce glycation, a process associated with diabetes.

- **Iron Absorption:** Pistachios' copper content aids in the absorption of iron from food sources.

Selection and Storage

When selecting pistachios, choose those that are:

- Compact and uniform in size

- Off-white in color

- Heavy in hand

- Free from cracks, mold, spots, and rancid smell

Store pistachios in an airtight container in a cool, dark place. Unshelled pistachios can last for several months, while shelled kernels should be refrigerated to prevent rancidity.

Culinary Uses

Pistachios are versatile ingredients that can be enjoyed in various ways:

- **Snacking:** Pistachios can be eaten on their own, roasted, or salted.

- **Salads:** Crushed pistachios add a nutty crunch to salads.

- **Desserts:** Pistachios are a common ingredient in baklava, ice cream, and other desserts.

- **Baking:** Pistachios can be incorporated into biscuits, cakes, and other baked goods.

Conclusion

Pistachios are a nutritional powerhouse, offering a wealth of health benefits and culinary versatility. Their rich nutrient profile, unique flavor, and crunchy texture make them a valuable addition to a balanced diet.

Chapter Fourteen

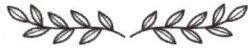

Walnuts – Natural Goodness

The walnut tree, scientifically known as *Juglans regia*, is a large, deciduous tree native to Central Asia and the Middle East. It has been cultivated for centuries for its edible nuts, which are a popular snack and ingredient in various culinary creations. Walnuts are not only delicious but also offer a wealth of health benefits due to their rich nutrient content.

Botanical Characteristics

Walnut trees are typically 30-50 feet tall, with a broad, spreading canopy and dark green leaves. They are monoecious, meaning that each tree produces both male and female flowers. The male flowers are long, catkin-like structures, while the female flowers are small and greenish.

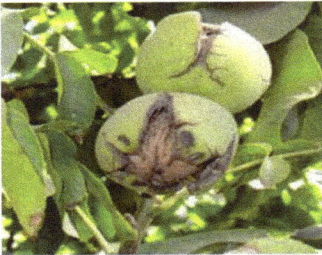

Walnuts Fruit

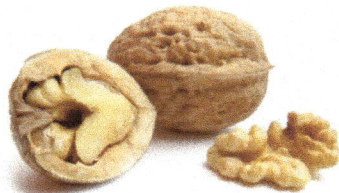

Walnuts

Cultivation and Production

Walnut trees are primarily grown in temperate regions worldwide, with major producers including China, India, the United States,

Turkey, and Iran. They thrive in well-drained, fertile soils and require ample sunlight. Walnut trees are typically propagated by grafting, a technique that involves joining a scion (the desired variety) to a rootstock (a hardy root system). Grafting allows for the propagation of desired characteristics and faster growth.

Nutritional Profile

Walnuts are a nutritional powerhouse, packed with essential nutrients that contribute to overall health. They are an excellent source of:

- **Healthy Fats:** Walnuts are particularly rich in omega-3 fatty acids, especially alpha-linolenic acid (ALA), which plays a crucial role in heart health and brain function.

- **Protein:** Walnuts provide a significant amount of protein, making them a valuable plant-based source of this essential nutrient.

- **Fiber:** Walnuts are a good source of dietary fiber, which aids in digestion, promotes gut health, and contributes to satiety.

- **Vitamins and Minerals:** Walnuts are a rich source of vitamins E, B complex vitamins, and minerals such as magnesium, manganese, copper, and phosphorus.

Walnut oil offers several beneficial properties that contribute to overall health and well-being:

- Improved blood circulation

- Reduced heart disease risk

- Anti-inflammatory effects

- Hormone balance

- Improved skin health

- Eczema prevention

- Anti-aging properties

Health Benefits

Regular consumption of walnuts has been associated with a range of health benefits, including:

- **Heart Health:** The omega-3 fatty acids in walnuts may help lower LDL (bad) cholesterol and raise HDL (good) cholesterol levels, reducing the risk of heart disease.

- **Brain Health:** The omega-3 fatty acids and antioxidants in walnuts may help protect brain function and reduce the risk of neurodegenerative diseases like Alzheimer's and Parkinson's.

- **Weight Management:** Walnuts' high protein, fiber, and healthy fat content promote satiety and may aid in weight management.

- **Inflammation Reduction:** The antioxidants and omega-3 fatty acids in walnuts may help reduce chronic inflammation, which is linked to various health conditions.

- **Diabetes Management:** Walnuts may help improve blood sugar control and reduce the risk of type 2 diabetes.

Culinary Uses

Walnuts are versatile ingredients that add a nutty flavor and crunchy texture to various culinary creations. They are commonly enjoyed as a snack, either on their own or roasted and salted. Walnuts are also frequently used in:

- **Baked Goods:** Walnuts add a rich flavor and texture to cakes, cookies, breads, and other pastries.

- **Salads and Savory Dishes:** Crushed walnuts add a nutty crunch to salads, vegetable dishes, and cheese plates.

- **Sauces and Dressings:** Walnuts are often used in pesto, a classic Italian sauce, and can also be incorporated into salad dressings and marinades.

- **Non-Dairy Milk and Cheese Alternatives:** Walnuts can be used to make nutritious dairy-free milk and cheese alternatives.

Selection and Storage

When selecting walnuts, choose those that are:

- Heavy in hand

- Free from cracks or blemishes

- Have a pleasant nutty aroma

- Store walnuts in an airtight container in a cool, dark place. Shelled walnuts can last for several months, while unshelled walnuts can last up to a year.

Conclusion

Walnuts are a nutrient-dense food with a wide range of health benefits. Their rich flavor, crunchy texture, and versatility in various culinary applications make them a valuable addition to a balanced diet. Incorporating walnuts into your regular diet can contribute to overall health and well-being.

Walnut oil is a versatile and beneficial substance with numerous applications in personal care, health, and various industries. Its therapeutic properties, nutritional value, and culinary versatility make it a valuable addition to a balanced lifestyle.

Chapter Fifteen

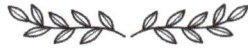

Continental Nuts: Global Delights

The world of nuts is a diverse and fascinating one, filled with an abundance of flavors, textures, and nutritional benefits. While some nuts are widely known and commercially available, such as almonds, cashews, walnuts, and peanuts, there exists a hidden realm of rare continental nuts, indigenous to specific continents or regions and relatively less common. Embark on a global nutty adventure as we explore these unique gems of the plant kingdom.

Acorn's Nut: The Oak Tree's Treasure

Nestled amidst the branches of towering oak trees lies the acorn's nut, a treasure trove of nutrients and a testament to nature's ingenuity. Found all over the world, acorns have been a staple food source for many cultures for millennia, revered for their rich flavor and nutritional value.

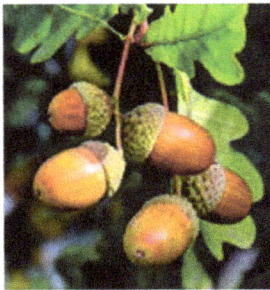

Acorn's Nut on Tree

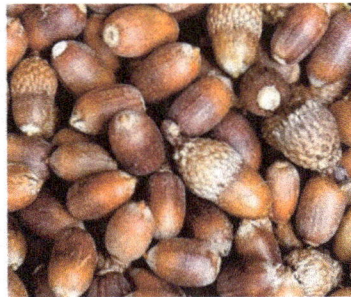

Acorn's Nut out of Pod

Acorns are high in carbohydrates, protein, and fiber, providing a substantial source of energy for those who consume them. They also contain essential minerals like potassium, magnesium, and calcium, playing a crucial role in maintaining overall health. However, acorns also harbor tannins, compounds that impart a bitter taste and make them difficult to digest. To overcome this hurdle, traditional methods involve soaking, boiling, or roasting acorns before consumption.

Indigenous peoples in North America and Europe have a long history of utilizing acorns as a food source. Native American tribes incorporated acorns into their diet, creating bread, soups, and other culinary creations. In Europe, acorns served as a substitute for wheat during times of scarcity, providing sustenance during challenging periods.

Today, acorns are less commonly consumed, but their nutritional value and unique flavor continue to captivate enthusiasts. They are sometimes used in animal feed and even serve as an alternative to coffee beans. Overall, acorns stand as a testament to the adaptability and ingenuity of nature, offering a nutritious and versatile food source that has enriched many cultures throughout history.

As we venture further into the realm of rare continental nuts, we discover a kaleidoscope of flavors and textures, each with its unique story to tell. Join us as we explore these hidden gems and uncover their culinary and nutritional wonders.

Atherton Oak Nut: A Tropical Treasure

Nestled amidst the lush rainforests of the Atherton Tablelands in Queensland, Australia, lies a natural treasure – the Atherton Oak Nut. This unique seed pod, with its distinctive shape and spiky projections, has captivated artists and craftspeople alike, becoming a prized material for intricate sculptures and decorative objects.

The Atherton Oak Nut, the fruit of the Lithocarpus densiflorus tree, is a native of Southeast Asia and the Pacific Islands. It has found a home in the Atherton Tablelands, where its rough exterior belies a treasure trove of edible nuts. These small kernels boast a delightful sweetness and nutty flavor, adding a touch of the tropics to any culinary creation.

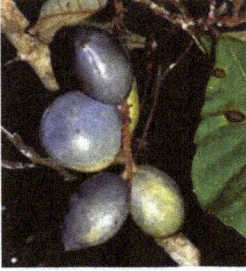

Atherton Oak Nut on Tree   Artherton Oak nut in and out of shell

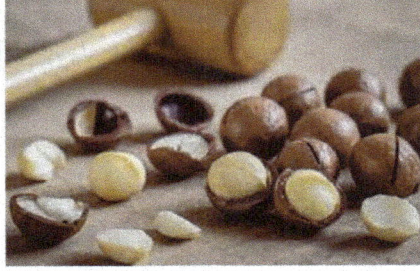

Despite its culinary potential, the Atherton Oak Nut has gained prominence more for its aesthetic appeal than its gastronomic qualities. Its spherical form, adorned with sharp, spiky projections, has inspired artists like Gabi Sturman to create mesmerizing sculptures that capture the essence of the rainforest's intricate beauty.

Woodworkers and craftspeople also find themselves drawn to the Atherton Oak Nut's unique texture and durability. Its hard shell and spiky exterior pose a challenge to those seeking to extract the edible nuts within, but for artists, this challenge becomes an opportunity to transform the natural material into works of art.

The Atherton Oak Nut stands as a testament to the ingenuity of nature, offering not only a source of sustenance but also a canvas for creativity. Its unique shape, texture, and versatility have made it a sought-after material in the art world, showcasing the boundless inspiration that nature provides. As we continue to explore the natural world, we uncover hidden gems like the Atherton Oak Nut, reminding us of the wonders that await those who venture beyond the ordinary.

Baru Nut: A Brazilian Treasure with Global Appeal

Emerging from the heart of Brazil's Cerrado region lies a nutritional gem, the Baru nut, also known as the Barukas Nut or "Brazilian almond." This remarkable nut, harvested from the towering Baruzeiro tree, has captivated taste buds and health enthusiasts alike, earning its place as a sought-after culinary delight and a nutritional powerhouse.

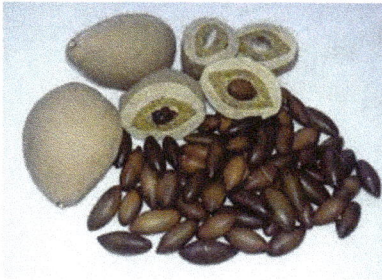

Baru Nut with Pod Exposed   Baru Nut Out of Pod

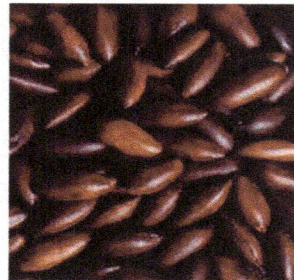

The Baru nut's allure lies in its delicate balance of taste and texture. Its mild, subtly sweet flavor entices the palate, while its crunchy texture provides a satisfying contrast. This symphony of flavors makes it a versatile ingredient, gracing both sweet and savory creations.

Beyond its captivating taste, the Baru nut boasts an impressive nutritional profile. It is a rich source of healthy fats, providing the body with essential fatty acids that support various bodily functions. Its abundance of protein and fiber contributes to satiety and overall well-being. Additionally, the Baru nut is brimming with vitamins and minerals, including vitamin E, magnesium, and zinc, all of which play crucial roles in maintaining optimal health.

In Brazil, the Baru nut is a culinary staple, seamlessly integrated into both sweet and savory dishes. Locals savor its raw form, enjoying its natural crunch and delicate flavor. Roasting enhances its nutty aroma and intensifies its taste, making it a popular addition to salads, desserts, and trail mixes. Baru nut oil, prized for its nutty flavor and high smoke point, is a culinary staple in Brazilian kitchens, adding a touch of sophistication to various dishes.

The Baru nut's fame has transcended borders, gaining popularity worldwide due to its unique taste and nutritional benefits. Health-conscious individuals embrace it as a healthy snack alternative to other nuts, incorporating it into their diets to reap its nutritional rewards. Food manufacturers recognize its potential, incorporating it into a range of healthy products, such as energy bars and granola, catering to the growing demand for wholesome, nutritious options.

The Baru nut stands as a testament to the bounty of nature, offering not only a culinary delight but also a treasure trove of essential nutrients. Its delicate flavor, crunchy texture, and impressive nutritional profile have made it a sought-after ingredient, gracing tables and energizing bodies worldwide. As we continue to explore the wonders of nature, we uncover gems like the Baru nut, reminding us of the vast array of culinary and nutritional treasures that await discovery.

Beech Nut: A Forgotten Forage with Enduring Value

Nestled amidst the boughs of towering beech trees, a humble treasure lies hidden – the beech nut. This small, unassuming fruit, often overlooked in the modern world, holds a rich history and a wealth of nutritional benefits, making it a worthy addition to our culinary and health repertoire.

Indigenous cultures have long recognized the beech nut's value as a food source, incorporating it into their diets for centuries. Its versatility allowed for various preparation methods, from roasting and boiling to grinding into flour for baking. Beech nuts were not merely sustenance; they were a cherished resource, providing essential nutrients and a unique flavor profile.

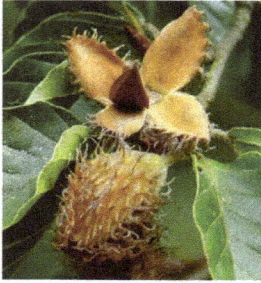

Beech Nut on Tree   Beech Nut Out of Pod

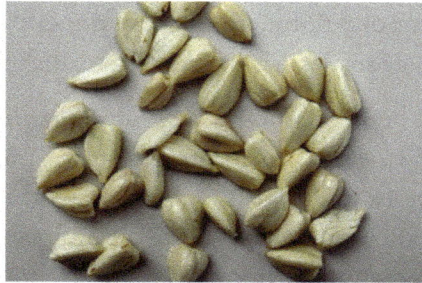

Despite its historical significance, the beech nut has faded into obscurity in many parts of the world. Commercialization and the availability of more widely known nuts have overshadowed its presence. Yet, a resurgence of interest in wild foods and a renewed appreciation for traditional ingredients are bringing the beech nut back into the spotlight.

Beech nuts offer an impressive nutritional profile, boasting protein, fiber, and healthy fats. They are also a rich source of vitamins and minerals, including vitamin E, manganese, and magnesium, essential for maintaining overall health and well-being. Their antioxidant properties further enhance their value, contributing to the body's defenses against oxidative stress and chronic diseases.

While not as readily available as their more popular counterparts, beech nuts can be found in specialty stores and farmers' markets, often at a fraction of the cost. Their subtle yet distinct flavor adds a unique dimension to various culinary creations. Ground into flour, they can enrich baked goods with a nutty, earthy undertone. Crushed, they provide a satisfying crunch to salads and desserts. Their versatility extends to flavorings and oils, imparting a delicate nutty essence to culinary creations.

In addition to their culinary applications, beech nuts have also gained recognition in the production of certain alcoholic beverages. Their fermentation imparts a unique flavor profile to spirits, adding complexity and depth to these libations.

The beech nut, once a staple in the diets of indigenous cultures, now stands as a forgotten forage with enduring value. Its nutritional richness, culinary versatility, and historical significance make it a worthy addition to our modern food landscape. As we rediscover the treasures of the natural world, the beech nut emerges as a reminder of the simple, wholesome goodness that nature has to offer.

Betel Nut - (areca nut)

Betel nut is a seed of the Areca palm tree, scientifically known as Areca catechu. It is commonly chewed in many parts of South and Southeast Asia, the Pacific Islands, and East Africa as a mild stimulant.

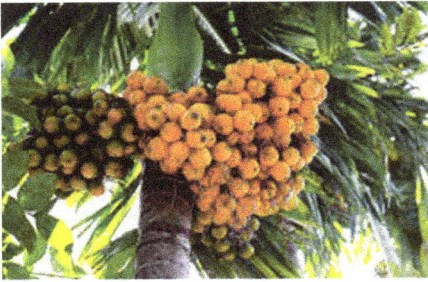

Betel Nut on Tree

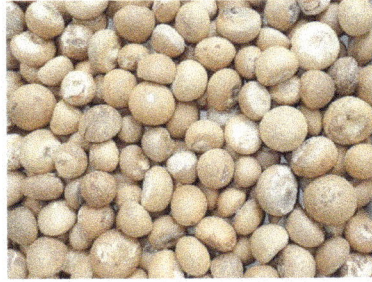

Betel Nut Out on Shell

Betel nut is usually wrapped in a betel leaf with lime and sometimes mixed with other ingredients, such as tobacco, spices, and sweeteners. When chewed, it produces a mild buzz and can have effects like caffeine, including increased alertness and heightened mood.

However, betel nut use is associated with various health risks. The nut contains arecoline, a chemical that can lead to addiction, oral cancer, and other health problems. Long-term use of betel nut can also lead to tooth decay, gum disease, and staining of the teeth and mouth.

Despite the health risks, betel nut is deeply ingrained in the cultural and social practices of many communities, particularly in South Asia. It is often used in traditional ceremonies, social gatherings, and religious rituals.

Black Walnut: A North American Treasure

Standing tall amidst the landscapes of North America, particularly in the eastern United States, is the majestic Black Walnut tree (Juglans nigra), a testament to nature's ingenuity and a source of valuable resources. Its towering presence, reaching heights of up to 100 feet, is complemented by a thick, furrowed bark that bears witness to its enduring spirit.

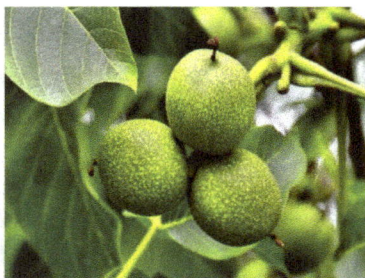

Black Walnut on Tree

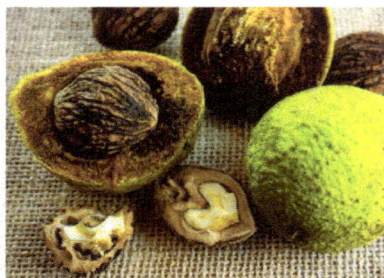

Black Walnut in Open Pod

The Black Walnut's elegance extends beyond its stature, as it adorns its branches with alternate, compound leaves, their pinnately lobed structure and dark green hue painting a captivating scene against the sky. Its reproductive cycle is equally captivating, with separate male and female flowers, the male flowers forming long, drooping catkins and the female flowers appearing in small clusters.

From these delicate blossoms emerges the tree's prized possession – the Black Walnut. Encased in a thick, hard outer shell, this treasure trove of nutrients boasts a bold, nutty flavor that has captivated palates for centuries. Its richness in protein, fiber, healthy fats, and minerals like manganese, magnesium, and phosphorus makes it a nutritional powerhouse, eagerly sought after for its culinary versatility.

Black Walnut's contributions extend beyond the dining table, as its wood has long been revered for its strength, durability, and aesthetic appeal. Its dark brown color and rich, warm grain pattern make it a prized material for furniture makers, flooring specialists, and woodworkers of all levels, transforming it into exquisite pieces that grace homes and businesses alike.

However, the Black Walnut's presence is not without its complexities. Its leaves, bark, and roots contain a chemical called juglone, which can be toxic to certain plant species, limiting the growth of other flora in its vicinity. Additionally, its dense shade and deep roots can pose challenges for other plants struggling to thrive under its imposing canopy.

Despite these potential drawbacks, the Black Walnut remains a valuable asset to the ecosystem, providing habitat for a variety of wildlife and contributing to the overall biodiversity of the landscape. Its resilience, adaptability, and unique combination of culinary and aesthetic qualities make it a true North American treasure, a testament to the remarkable diversity and balance of nature.

Bunya Nut: A Culinary and Cultural Gem of Australia

Emerging from the heart of Australia's lush rainforests, the Bunya nut stands as a culinary and cultural treasure, deeply interwoven with the history and traditions of indigenous peoples. Harvested from the towering Bunya pine tree, this remarkable nut has nourished and enriched the lives of Australians for millennia.

The Bunya pine tree, a majestic evergreen sentinel of the Australian landscape, can reach heights of up to 50 meters and live for over a thousand years. Its crown shelters and nurtures the Bunya nut, a culinary gem encased in a protective pod. These large nuts, weighing up to 4 kilograms each, hold a treasure trove of nutrients and a unique flavor profile.

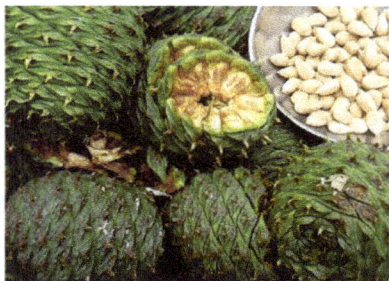

Bunya Nut In Pod   Bunya Nut Out Of Pod

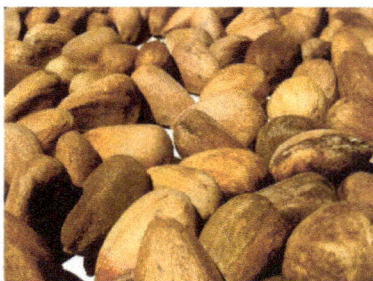

For thousands of years, the Bunya nut has been a cornerstone of indigenous Australian cuisine. Its rich protein, fiber, and essential nutrients, including potassium, magnesium, and iron, provided sustenance and vitality to indigenous communities. The nuts' high antioxidant content further enhanced their value, offering protection against cellular damage caused by free radicals.

The versatility of the Bunya nut extends beyond its nutritional prowess. Its unique flavor and texture, a symphony of nutty richness and satisfying crunch, have captivated palates for generations. The nuts can be enjoyed raw, roasted, or boiled, each preparation method revealing a distinct dimension of their culinary essence.

Indigenous Australian cuisine embraces the Bunya nut, incorporating it into traditional dishes such as stews and soups. Its hearty presence enriches these culinary creations, adding depth and complexity to the flavors. Today, the Bunya nut continues to inspire modern Australian chefs, who incorporate it into their innovative dishes, showcasing its versatility and adaptability.

The Bunya nut's significance extends beyond its culinary applications, as it holds deep cultural and spiritual value for many indigenous peoples. The Bunya tree is a sacred symbol, revered for its generosity and its role in maintaining the balance of the natural world.

Every three years, the Bunya pine tree produces a bountiful harvest, triggering the Bunya festival, a grand celebration of this natural treasure. Indigenous communities gather to partake in the bounty, sharing meals, exchanging stories, and reaffirming their connection to the land and its gifts.

The Bunya nut, a culinary and cultural gem, stands as a testament to the enduring relationship between indigenous Australians and the natural world. Its nutritional richness, culinary versatility, and deep cultural significance make it a valuable symbol of Australia's unique heritage. As we continue to explore the wonders of this land, we uncover treasures like the Bunya nut, reminding us of the profound connections that exist between humanity and nature.

Breadnut: A Tropical Treasure with Culinary and Nutritional Promise

Emerging from the lush rainforests of New Guinea, the Maluku Islands, and the Philippines lies a tropical treasure – the breadnut, a close relative of the breadfruit. This versatile fruit, known for its starchy flesh and unique flavor, offers a wealth of culinary possibilities and nutritional benefits.

The breadnut, the wild ancestor of the breadfruit, bears a striking resemblance to its descendant, sharing a similar appearance and growth pattern. It is a medium-sized tree that can produce up to 800 fruits per year, each weighing around 800 grams. Its green skin encases a starchy, potato-like flesh that, when cooked, takes on a mild, slightly sweet flavor.

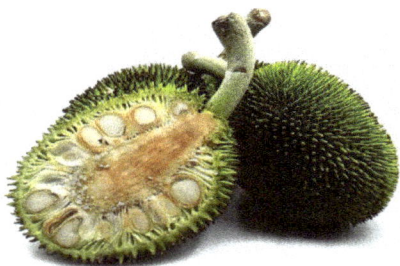

Breadnut From Tree

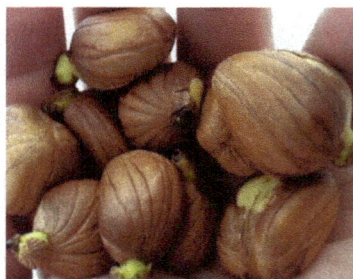

Breadnut Out of Pod

Breadnut's culinary versatility shines through its adaptability to various cooking methods. Whether boiled, baked, fried, or roasted, the breadnut readily lends itself to a range of dishes, adding a satisfying texture and a subtly sweet undertone to savory creations and desserts alike.

Beyond its culinary appeal, the breadnut boasts an impressive nutritional profile. It is a rich source of carbohydrates, fiber, and essential vitamins and minerals, including vitamin C, potassium, and magnesium. Its low fat and cholesterol content further enhances its nutritional value, making it a potentially beneficial addition to a balanced diet.

Breadnut plays a significant role in traditional cuisine, particularly in regions where it is native. In various cultures, the breadnut is mashed, fermented, or dried to produce flour, which serves as a versatile ingredient for bread, cakes, and other culinary creations.

While the breadnut's raw form is not typically consumed due to its starchy nature and lack of sweetness, cooking transforms its texture and flavor, making it a palatable and nutritious addition to meals. Its versatility extends beyond its culinary applications, as it is also used in traditional medicine to treat various ailments, including rheumatoid arthritis, digestive issues, and skin conditions.

The breadnut, a tropical treasure with culinary and nutritional promise, stands as a testament to the bounty of nature. Its unique flavor, starchy texture, and impressive nutritional profile make it a valuable ingredient in both traditional and modern cuisine. As we continue to explore the world's diverse flora, we uncover gems like the breadnut, reminding us of the vast array of culinary delights and nutritional riches that nature has to offer.

Butternut: A North American Treasure with Culinary and Nutritional Appeal

Emerging from the heart of North America's forests, the butternut, also known as the white walnut, stands as a culinary gem, captivating palates with its rich, buttery flavor and offering a wealth of nutritional benefits. This remarkable nut, nestled within a hard, woody shell and encased in a green, fleshy husk, has long been a staple in traditional cuisine and continues to inspire modern culinary creations.

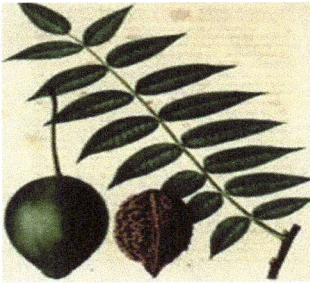

Butter Nut Pod Green and Dried   Butter Nut (White Walnut) in Open Pod

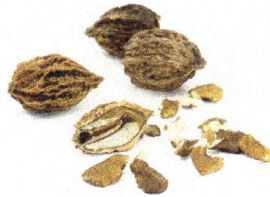

Upon reaching maturity, the butternut's husk transforms from vibrant green to a warm, inviting brown, signaling the nut's readiness to reveal its delectable treasure. The nut itself, adorned with intricate markings, holds a symphony of flavors, its buttery richness complemented by subtle hints of earthiness and sweetness.

This culinary gem seamlessly integrates into a diverse range of culinary creations. Butternut's versatility shines through in its adaptability to both sweet and savory dishes. In the realm of baking, it lends its unique flavor and texture to breads, pies, and other baked goods, adding a touch of elegance to every bite.

Savory creations also welcome the butternut's presence, as it enriches soups and stews with its depth of flavor and satisfying texture. Ground into a paste or butter, it transforms into a versatile spread or topping, adding a touch of sophistication to various dishes. Butternut oil, extracted from the nuts, further extends its culinary reach, serving as a natural flavoring or an ingredient in skincare products.

Beyond its culinary versatility, the butternut boasts an impressive nutritional profile, making it a valuable addition to a balanced diet. It is a rich source of protein, providing essential amino acids for bodily functions. Its abundance of healthy fats supports the body's energy production and contributes to overall well-being.

Dietary fiber, an essential component of a healthy diet, is generously supplied by the butternut, aiding in digestion and promoting gut health. Vitamins and minerals, including vitamin E, magnesium, and potassium, further enhance the butternut's nutritional value, contributing to various bodily processes and maintaining overall health.

The butternut's significance extends beyond its culinary and nutritional attributes, as it holds a prominent place in the cultural landscape of North America. Indigenous cultures have long revered the butternut, incorporating it into their traditional practices and recognizing its medicinal properties.

Today, the butternut continues to captivate the hearts and palates of those fortunate enough to encounter it. Its unique flavor, culinary versatility, and impressive nutritional profile have solidified its place as a North American treasure, a testament to the bounty of nature and the ingenuity of those who have embraced its culinary and medicinal gifts. As we continue to explore the wonders of the natural world, we uncover gems like the butternut, reminding us of the vast array of culinary delights and nutritional riches that await discovery.

Cedar Nut: A Culinary and Medicinal Gem from the Siberian Taiga

Deep within the vast expanse of the Siberian taiga, amidst the towering Siberian cedar trees, lies a culinary and medicinal gem – the cedar nut. These small, elongated nuts, encased in a hard, woody shell, hold a treasure trove of flavor, nutrients, and potential health benefits.

Cedar nuts, the seeds of the Siberian cedar tree, have long been revered for their unique flavor profile, often described as a harmonious blend of nutty, earthy, and slightly sweet notes. Their versatility in the kitchen is undeniable, seamlessly transitioning from sweet to savory creations.

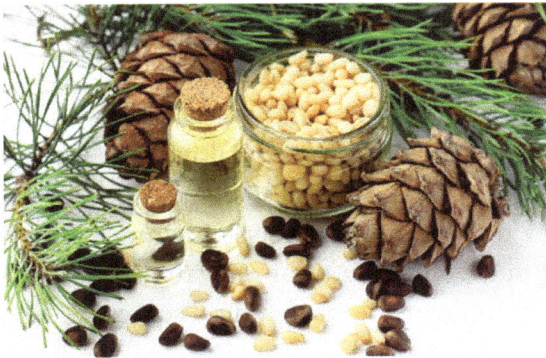

Cedar Nut in and out of pod, and it's oil

In the realm of desserts, cedar nuts grace cakes, pastries, and cookies, adding a delightful crunch and a subtle hint of their distinctive flavor. Their richness complements the sweetness of these creations, creating a symphony of textures and tastes that tantalize the palate.

Savory dishes also embrace the cedar nut's versatility. Stews and salads welcome its presence, as the nuts infuse them with a depth of flavor and a satisfying crunch, transforming these culinary creations into gourmet experiences. Cedar nut oil, extracted from the nuts, further enhances the culinary landscape, serving as a cooking oil, salad dressing, and condiment, imparting its unique flavor and nutritional value to various dishes.

Beyond their culinary applications, cedar nuts hold a prominent place in traditional medicine and natural remedies. The oil extracted from these remarkable nuts is believed to possess a range of health benefits, including anti-inflammatory and antioxidant properties, making it a valuable addition to natural healing practices.

Indigenous cultures have long recognized the cedar nut's medicinal potential, incorporating it into their traditional remedies to address digestive issues, respiratory problems, and skin conditions. The nuts' reputation for promoting overall health and well-being has endured through the ages, a testament to their inherent value.

Cedar nuts, a culinary and medicinal gem from the Siberian taiga, stand as a symbol of nature's enduring bounty and the profound connection between humanity and the natural world. Their unique flavor, culinary versatility, and potential health benefits make them a valuable addition to both traditional and modern diets and practices. As we continue to explore the wonders of nature, we uncover treasures like the cedar nut, reminding us of the vast array of culinary delights and potential health remedies that await discovery.

Candle Nut: A Polynesian Gem with Culinary, Medicinal, and Cosmetic Appeal

Emerging from the lush rainforests of Southeast Asia and the Pacific Islands, the candle nut, also known as the kukui nut or Indian walnut, stands as a culinary, medicinal, and cosmetic gem, deeply interwoven with the cultural heritage of Polynesian communities. This remarkable nut, encased in a hard, spherical shell, holds a wealth of flavor, nutrients, and potential health benefits.

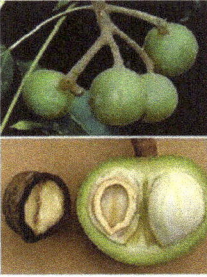

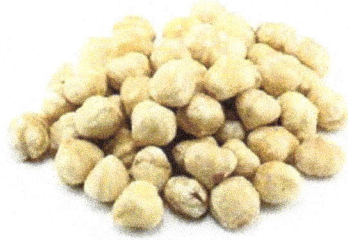

Candle Nut On tree and in Pod   Candle Nut Out of Pod

Candle nuts, harvested from the towering candle nut tree, have long been a staple in Polynesian cuisine, particularly in Hawaii, where they are revered as a symbol of enlightenment, protection, and peace. Their rich, nutty flavor, reminiscent of macadamia nuts, seamlessly integrates into a variety of dishes, from savory creations to sweet indulgences.

Roasted or boiled, candle nuts lend a satisfying crunch and a depth of flavor to salads, stews, and stir-fries. Their versatility extends to sweet treats, where they grace cakes, pastries, and desserts with their unique nutty undertone. The oil extracted from the candle nut, known as kukui nut oil, is a prized cooking oil, valued for its high smoke point and delicate nutty flavor.

Beyond its culinary applications, the candle nut holds significant medicinal value. Traditional Polynesian medicine has long utilized candle nuts to treat a range of ailments, including skin conditions, headaches, and digestive issues. Modern research suggests that candle nuts may also possess anti-inflammatory and anti-cancer properties, further solidifying their reputation as a natural remedy.

The cosmetic industry has also embraced the candle nut's potential. The oil extracted from the nut is rich in fatty acids, making it a valuable ingredient in moisturizing creams, lotions, and hair care products. Its ability to nourish and protect the skin has earned it a prominent place in Polynesian beauty practices.

Candle nuts, a Polynesian gem with culinary, medicinal, and cosmetic appeal, epitomize the deep connection between humanity and the natural world. Their unique flavor, nutritional profile, and potential health benefits have made them a vital component of Polynesian culture, a testament to the enduring bounty that nature provides. As we continue to explore the wonders of the world's diverse ecosystems, we uncover treasures like the candle nut, reminding us of the vast array of culinary delights, medicinal remedies, and natural beauty solutions that await discovery.

Cocoa: A Culinary and Health Treasure from the Tropical Rainforests

Emerging from the lush rainforests of the Americas, cocoa, also known as cacao, stands as a culinary and health treasure, captivating palates with its rich, chocolaty flavor and offering a wealth of potential health benefits. This remarkable plant, with its vibrant green leaves and striking red or yellow pods, holds a treasure trove of delectable beans that have transformed culinary traditions and inspired countless creations.

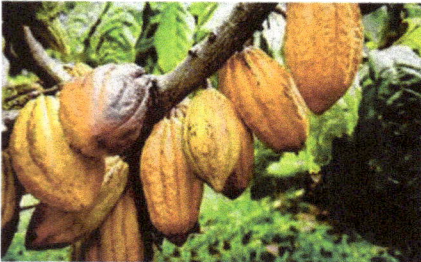

Cocoa On Tree on Pod   Cocoa Open of Pod and Dried Beens

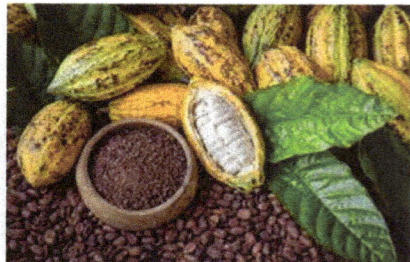

Cocoa's flavor profile is a symphony of complexity, boasting a deep, chocolaty richness complemented by subtle hints of bitterness, earthiness, and sweetness. Its versatility in the kitchen is unparalleled, seamlessly transitioning from sweet to savory dishes and lending its unique flavor to a vast array of culinary creations.

In the realm of desserts, cocoa reigns supreme. Its rich, indulgent flavor graces cakes, pastries, and chocolates, transforming them into delectable treats that tantalize the senses. Cocoa powder, the finely ground form of the beans, lends its magic to brownies, cookies, and other baked goods, adding a touch of decadence to every bite.

Savory creations also welcome cocoa's presence. Its subtle bitterness and earthy undertones enhance the flavors of sauces, marinades, and stews, adding depth and complexity to culinary masterpieces. Cocoa chili, a traditional dish from Mesoamerica, showcases the harmonious blend of cocoa's rich flavor with the spicy warmth of chili peppers.

Beyond its culinary applications, cocoa holds a prominent place in traditional medicine and natural remedies. Its rich content of antioxidants, flavonoids, and other beneficial compounds has been linked to numerous health benefits, including reducing inflammation, improving heart health, and boosting brain function.

Indigenous cultures have long revered cocoa for its medicinal properties, incorporating it into their traditional practices to address a range of ailments. The beans have been used to treat coughs, fever, and fatigue, and modern research continues to explore the potential of cocoa to promote overall well-being.

In recent years, there has been a growing movement towards ethical and sustainable cocoa production. Consumers are increasingly seeking out fair trade and organic cocoa products, driven by a desire to ensure fair wages and sustainable farming practices for cocoa farmers in developing countries.

Overall, cocoa stands as a versatile and valuable plant that has played an integral role in many cultures throughout history. Its rich flavor, potential health benefits, and cultural significance make it a beloved and enduring ingredient in countless cuisines and products. As we continue to explore the wonders of the natural world, we uncover treasures like cocoa, reminding us of the vast array of culinary delights, potential health benefits, and the importance of ethical and sustainable practices

Ginkgo Nut:

Ginkgo nut, also known as ginkgo biloba, is the seed of the ginkgo tree, a living fossil that has been around for more than 200 million years. The nut has a hard, yellowish-green shell and is about the size of a grape. Ginkgo nuts are native to China, Japan, and Korea, and have been used in traditional medicine for thousands of years.

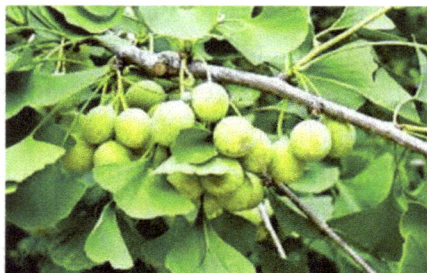

Ginkgo Nut on Tree

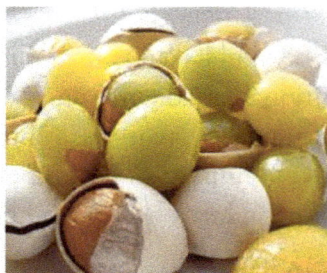

Ginkgo Nut Out of Pod

Ginkgo nuts are a rich source of antioxidants, flavonoids, and other beneficial compounds that have been linked to numerous health benefits. They are also a good source of protein, fiber, and essential vitamins and minerals, including iron, zinc, and vitamin E.

In traditional Chinese medicine, ginkgo nuts are used to treat a variety of ailments, including asthma, coughs, and digestive disorders. They are also believed to improve memory and cognitive function, and to have a calming effect on the nervous system.

In addition to their medicinal properties, ginkgo nuts are used in cooking and baking in China, Japan, and Korea. They have a slightly sweet, nutty flavor and can be roasted or boiled before being eaten.

Ginkgo nut soup and congee are popular dishes in Chinese cuisine, while ginkgo nuts are used to make a sweet dessert soup in Korea.

While ginkgo nuts are generally safe for most people to eat in moderation, they can cause allergic reactions in some individuals. In addition, raw nuts contain a toxic substance that can cause vomiting and other symptoms if eaten in large quantities.

Overall, ginkgo nuts are a unique and valuable food that have been used for thousands of years in traditional medicine and culinary traditions. Their rich flavor and potential health benefits make them a popular ingredient in many different dishes and products.

Hickory Nut

Hickory nut is a type of nut that comes from hickory trees, which are found in many parts of North America. The hickory nut is known for its rich, buttery flavor and is often used in cooking and baking.

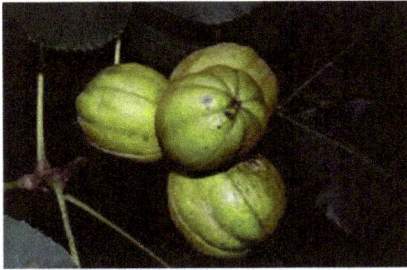

Hickory Nut On Tree   Hickory Nut Pod With Nut

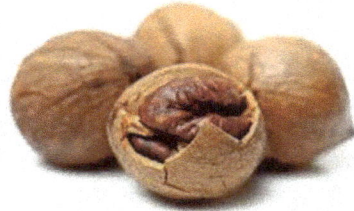

Hickory nuts are high in healthy fats, protein, and fiber, as well as vitamins and minerals such as vitamin E, magnesium, and zinc. They are also a good source of antioxidants, which can help protect against oxidative stress and reduce the risk of chronic diseases.

In North America, hickory nuts are commonly used in a variety of dishes, including pies, cakes, and cookies. They can be eaten raw or roasted and can also be used as a topping for salads and desserts.

Hickory nuts are a nutritious and tasty ingredient that can be enjoyed in many ways. However, they are also high in calories and should be consumed in moderation, especially if you are watching your weight. It is also important to note that some people may be allergic to hickory nuts, so it is always a good idea to check with your doctor if you are unsure about consuming them.

Karuka Nut: A Nutritional Treasure from the Tropical Rainforests

Emerging from the verdant depths of Southeast Asia, Papua New Guinea, and the Pacific Islands lies a nutritional treasure – the karuka nut, a remarkable gift from the Pangium edule tree. This unique nut, encased in a spiny, football-sized fruit pod, holds a wealth of nutrients, a rich cultural heritage, and a culinary versatility that has captivated palates for centuries.

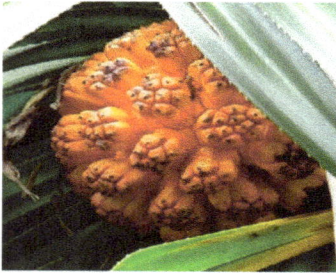

Karuka Pod On Tree

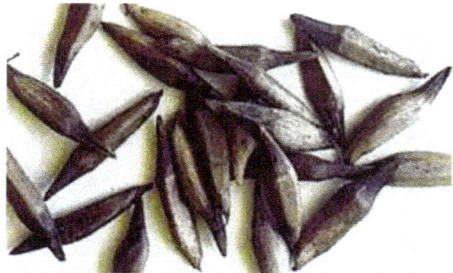

Karuka Nut Out of Pod

The karuka nut, revered for its high nutritional value, is a rich source of protein, providing essential amino acids for bodily functions. Its abundance of fiber aids in digestion, promotes gut health, and contributes to overall satiety. Vitamins and minerals, including vitamin C, iron, and calcium, further enhance its nutritional profile, supporting various bodily processes and maintaining overall well-being.

Karuka nuts, also known as pangium edule or kumpay nuts, have been a staple food source for thousands of years, deeply interwoven into the cultural fabric of many communities. Indigenous cultures have mastered the art of harvesting these precious nuts, traditionally climbing the tall Pangium edule trees and carefully removing the spiny fruit pods that hold the treasure within.

To prepare the nuts for consumption, a unique process is followed. The seeds are soaked in water for several days to remove any toxic compounds and then either boiled or roasted. Once prepared, the karuka nut reveals its culinary versatility, lending its unique flavor and texture to a diverse range of dishes.

In traditional cuisine, karuka nuts are often ground into flour and used to create a variety of dishes, from savory stews and soups to sweet puddings and pastries. Their rich, nutty flavor adds depth and complexity to culinary creations, while their nutritional value ensures a satisfying and wholesome meal.

Beyond its culinary applications, the karuka nut holds a prominent place in cultural traditions and rituals. In Papua New Guinea, the nuts play a significant role in the creation of intricate carvings, while in parts of Indonesia, they serve as a form of currency for trade. The karuka nut's cultural significance extends to celebrations and ceremonies, where its presence symbolizes abundance, prosperity, and interconnectedness with the natural world.

Overall, the karuka nut stands as a testament to the enduring bounty of nature and the profound connection between humanity and the natural world. Its nutritional richness, culinary versatility, and cultural significance make it a valuable addition to any diet and a symbol of the deep respect and appreciation for the gifts that nature provides. As we continue to explore the wonders of the world's diverse ecosystems, we uncover treasures like the karuka nut, reminding us of the vast array of nutritional riches and cultural gems that await discovery.

Kola Nut: A Stimulating Gem from West African Rainforests

Emerging from the heart of West Africa's lush rainforests, the kola nut, a caffeine-rich treasure, stands as a symbol of hospitality, a source of energy, and a testament to the enduring connection between humanity and the natural world. Encased within the star-shaped fruits of the kola tree, this remarkable nut holds a unique flavor, a wealth of potential health benefits, and a deep cultural significance that has shaped traditions for centuries.

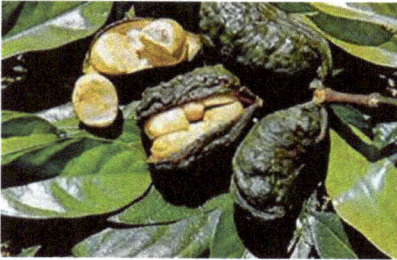

Kola Nut on Tree

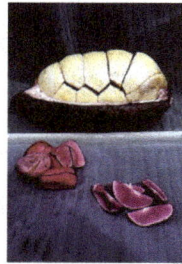

Kola Open Pod with Nuts

Kola nuts, harvested from the towering kola trees that can reach up to 20 meters tall, have long been revered for their stimulating properties. Their caffeine content, coupled with theobromine and other alkaloids, offers a boost in energy levels, enhancing alertness and promoting a sense of vitality. This invigorating effect has made kola nuts a cherished element of West African hospitality, traditionally offered to guests as a warm welcome and a symbol of respect.

Beyond their energizing properties, kola nuts have also been employed in traditional medicine for their potential health benefits. They are believed to aid in digestion, promoting gut health and easing digestive issues. Additionally, their antioxidant content suggests a role in protecting against oxidative stress, potentially reducing the risk of chronic diseases.

The kola nut's culinary applications extend beyond its traditional use as a stimulant. Its bitter taste and slightly astringent flavor add a unique dimension to beverages, often used to create kola-infused soft drinks and energy drinks. In some cultures, kola nuts are even ground into flour and incorporated into various culinary creations.

While kola nuts offer a range of potential benefits, it is crucial to exercise moderation in their consumption. Excessive intake can lead to negative side effects such as restlessness, anxiety, and heart palpitations. As with any caffeinated product, responsible consumption is key to unlocking the benefits of kola nuts without experiencing adverse effects.

The kola nut, a stimulating gem from West African rainforests, epitomizes the enduring bounty of nature and the profound connection between humanity and the natural world. Its invigorating properties, potential health benefits, and deep cultural significance make it a valuable addition to traditional practices and a testament to the wonders that nature holds. As we continue to explore the diverse ecosystems of our planet, we uncover treasures like the kola nut, reminding us of the vast array of natural gifts that await discovery.

Mongongo Nut: A Nutritious Treasure from the Kalahari Desert

Emerging from the heart of the vast Kalahari Desert, a remarkable treasure lies hidden within the sprawling mongongo tree – the mongongo nut, also known as the manketti nut. This nutrient-rich gem, encased in a sturdy, woody shell, holds a symphony of flavors and a wealth of nutritional benefits, making it a staple food and a vital part of the cultural heritage of southern Africa's indigenous communities.

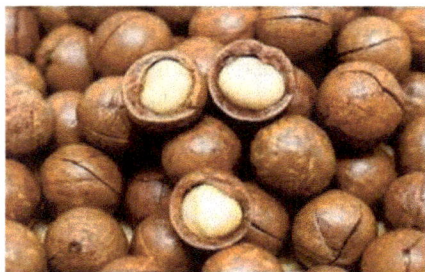

Mongongo Nut in Pod

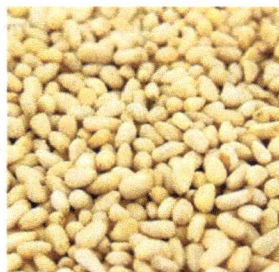

Mongongo Nut out of pod

Mongongo nuts, harvested from the majestic mongongo trees that can reach up to 20 meters tall, have long been revered for their unique flavor profile, often described as a harmonious blend of buttery richness and subtle hints of earthiness. Their versatility in the kitchen is undeniable, seamlessly transitioning from savory to sweet creations and adding a touch of culinary elegance to every bite.

In traditional cuisine, mongongo nuts grace porridge, stews, and sauces, lending their distinctive flavor and texture to these culinary masterpieces. Their rich, buttery undertones enhance the savory notes of these dishes, creating a symphony of flavors that tantalize the palate. The nuts are also ground into a delectable nut butter, a versatile ingredient that can be used as a spread, a flavor enhancer, or a base for nutritious smoothies.

Beyond their culinary applications, mongongo nuts hold a prominent place in traditional African medicine and cosmetics. The oil extracted from the nuts is believed to possess a range of healing properties, making it a valuable remedy for treating skin conditions like dryness and inflammation. Its natural protective properties have earned it a reputation as a natural sunscreen and insect repellent, safeguarding individuals against the harsh elements of the desert environment.

The mongongo nut, a nutritious treasure from the Kalahari Desert, stands as a testament to the enduring bounty of nature and the profound connection between humanity and the natural world. Its unique flavor, culinary versatility, and nutritional profile have made it an integral part of southern African culture and cuisine, a symbol of resilience, adaptability, and the profound respect for the gifts that nature provides. As we continue to explore the wonders of the world's diverse ecosystems, we uncover treasures like the mongongo nut, reminding us of the vast array of culinary delights, potential health benefits, and the importance of sustainable practices that preserve these natural treasures for future generations.

Nutmeg

Nutmeg is believed to have originated in the Banda Islands, which are part of present-day Indonesia. These islands, also known as the Spice Islands, have been a significant source of various valuable spices, including nutmeg, for centuries. Today, nutmeg is grown in several other countries as well, including Grenada, India, Malaysia, and Sri Lanka.

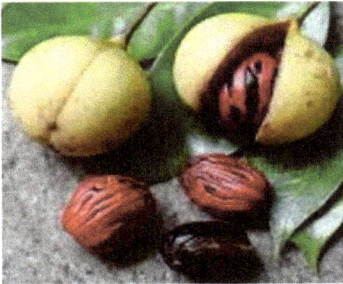

Nutmeg in and out of pod Tree

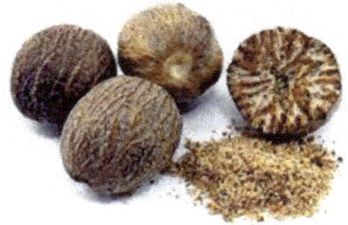

Nutmeg Out of Pod

Nutmeg is a spice that is commonly used in many cuisines and has been used for medicinal purposes for centuries. Nutmeg contains several nutrients and compounds that provide potential health benefits. Here are some of the health values associated with nutmeg:

1. Anti-inflammatory properties: Nutmeg contains compounds like myristicin and elemicin that have anti-inflammatory effects and may help to reduce inflammation in the body.

2. Digestive health: Nutmeg has traditionally been used to aid digestion and relieve stomach discomfort. It contains fiber, which helps to promote regular bowel movements.

3. Brain health: Nutmeg contains compounds that may improve cognitive function and memory. It may also have a calming effect and help to reduce anxiety.

4. Pain relief: Nutmeg has been used as a natural pain reliever for centuries. It contains compounds that may help to reduce pain and inflammation in the body.

5. Antioxidant properties: Nutmeg is rich in antioxidants, which help to protect cells from damage caused by free radicals.

It's important to note that consuming large amounts of nutmeg can be toxic and may cause hallucinations, nausea, and other health problems. So, it's best to use nutmeg in moderation as a spice in your food.

Clinical effects on the heart of nut meg

Nutmeg contains a compound called myristicin, which has been shown to have some effects on the heart. However, consuming large amounts of nutmeg can be toxic and may cause serious health problems, including cardiac effects.

In small amounts, nutmeg has been suggested to have potential benefits for the heart. For example, research suggests that myristicin may have antihypertensive properties, which means it may help to lower blood pressure. Additionally, some studies have suggested that nutmeg may have a positive effect on lipid levels, such as decreasing cholesterol levels, which can also be beneficial for heart health.

However, it's important to note that consuming large amounts of nutmeg can have negative effects on the heart. Ingesting high doses of nutmeg has been reported to cause tachycardia (a rapid heartbeat), palpitations, and even arrhythmias (abnormal heart rhythms). In some cases, these cardiac effects have been serious enough to require medical attention.

In summary, while nutmeg may have some potential benefits for heart health when consumed in small amounts, consuming large amounts can be dangerous and may cause serious health problems, including cardiac effects. As with any food or supplement, it's always best to consume nutmeg in moderation and talk to your doctor before using it for any specific health purposes.

Paradise Nut: A Culinary and Medicinal Gem from South American Rainforests

Emerging from the verdant depths of South American rainforests, the paradise nut, also known as the Sapucaia nut or the Castanha de Sapucaia, stands as a culinary and medicinal gem, captivating palates with its unique flavor and offering a wealth of potential health benefits. This remarkable nut, encased within the imposing fruit of the Lecythis pisonis tree, holds a symphony of flavors, a wealth of nutrients, and a rich cultural heritage that has captivated indigenous communities for centuries.

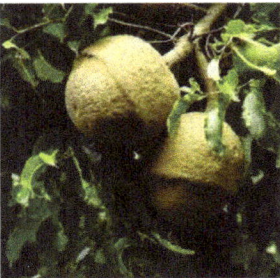

Paradise Nut in Pod on Tree

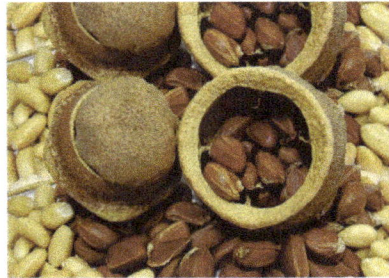

Paradise Nut in open pod and shelled

The paradise nut, adorned with a hard, outer shell, reveals its treasure upon cracking. The edible kernel, boasting a unique flavor often described as a blend of buttery richness, subtle earthiness, and hints of sweetness, has long been a coveted ingredient in traditional South American cuisine.

In culinary creations, paradise nuts seamlessly integrate into both savory and sweet dishes. Their rich, nutty flavor complements the hearty notes of stews and soups, while their subtle sweetness enhances the flavors of cakes, pastries, and other desserts. Paradise nut oil, extracted from the kernels, further extends the nut's culinary reach, serving as a versatile cooking oil, salad dressing, and ingredient in various recipes.

Beyond its culinary applications, the paradise nut holds a prominent place in traditional medicine. Indigenous cultures have long recognized its potential health benefits, incorporating it into their practices to address a range of ailments, including arthritis, inflammation, and digestive issues. The nut's anti-inflammatory properties and abundance of antioxidants contribute to its reputation as a natural remedy.

The paradise nut's cosmetic applications further expand its versatility. Its moisturizing properties have made it a valuable ingredient in soaps, lotions, and other beauty products, offering a natural way to nourish and protect the skin.

Harvesting paradise nuts is a challenging yet rewarding process. The towering Lecythis pisonis trees, reaching heights of up to 40 meters, pose a formidable obstacle, but the reward is well worth the effort. The nuts, often found at the very top of the trees, hold a unique flavor, a treasure trove of nutrients, and a rich cultural significance that makes them a prized commodity.

Overall, the paradise nut stands as a testament to the enduring bounty of nature and the profound connection between humanity and the natural world. Its unique flavor, culinary versatility, and potential health benefits make it a valuable addition to any diet and a symbol of the deep respect for the gifts that nature provides. As we continue to explore the wonders of the world's diverse ecosystems, we uncover treasures like the paradise nut, reminding us of the vast array of culinary delights, potential health benefits, and the importance of sustainable practices that preserve these natural treasures for future generations.

Pili Nut: A Treasure from the Philippine Islands

Nestled amidst the verdant landscapes of the Philippine Islands, a culinary and nutritional gem emerges from the towering pili tree – the pili nut, also known as the Canarium ovatum. This remarkable nut, enveloped in a hard, woody shell, holds a treasure trove of flavor, nutrients, and cultural significance, making it a cherished ingredient in Filipino cuisine and a symbol of the region's rich biodiversity.

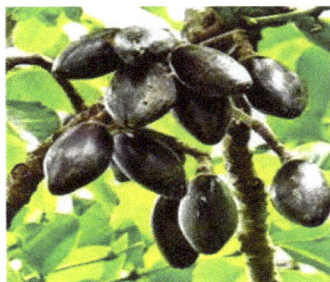

Pili Nut on Tree

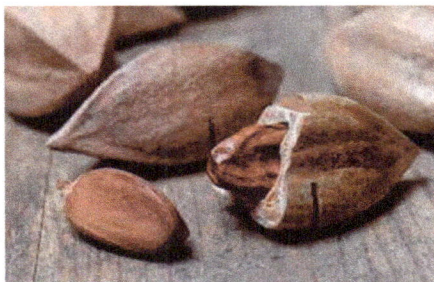

Pili Nut in and out of Pod

The pili nut, boasting a buttery texture and a delicate, slightly sweet flavor, has long been revered for its culinary versatility. Its rich, nutty undertones grace a variety of dishes, seamlessly transitioning from savory creations to sweet indulgences. In traditional Filipino cuisine, pili nuts are roasted and salted, offering a satisfying crunch and a depth of flavor that complements both savory and sweet dishes.

Pili nut oil, extracted from the kernels, further enhances the culinary landscape. Its high smoke point and mild flavor make it a versatile cooking oil, suitable for sautéing, stir-frying, and even baking. Its ability to impart a subtle nutty flavor to dishes without overwhelming the palate has made it a favorite among Filipino chefs.

Beyond its culinary applications, the pili nut holds a prominent place in Filipino culture. Its unique flavor and nutritional profile have earned it the moniker "King of Philippine Nuts," a testament to its esteemed status in the country's culinary heritage. Pili nuts are often incorporated into traditional celebrations, symbolizing abundance, prosperity, and a deep connection to the natural world.

The pili nut's nutritional value further solidifies its position as a dietary staple. Rich in healthy fats, protein, and fiber, it provides a sustained source of energy and essential nutrients. Its abundance of vitamins and minerals, including vitamin E, magnesium, and zinc, contributes to overall well-being and supports various bodily functions.

As the pili nut gains international recognition for its unique taste and nutritional benefits, it is finding its way into kitchens and health-conscious diets around the world. Its versatility as a snack, ingredient, and oil is opening doors to new culinary experiences and showcasing the Philippines' rich natural bounty.

Overall, the pili nut stands as a testament to the enduring connection between humanity and nature, a symbol of the Philippines' rich biodiversity and culinary heritage. Its unique flavor, nutritional profile, and cultural significance make it a valuable addition to any diet and a reminder of the vast array of culinary delights and potential health benefits that await discovery in the natural world.

Saba Nut: A South American Gem with Culinary and Nutritional Appeal

Emerging from the lush rainforests of Central and South America, the Saba nut, also known as the "monkey pot" or "apucaya nut," stands as a culinary and nutritional gem, deeply interwoven with the cultural heritage of indigenous communities. This remarkable nut, encased in a hard, woody shell, holds a unique flavor, a wealth of nutrients, and a variety of culinary applications that have captivated palates for centuries.

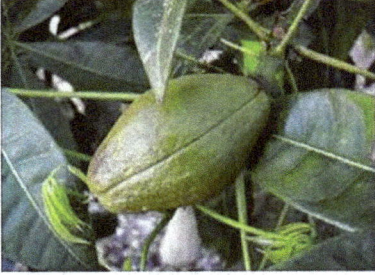

Saba Nut on Tree

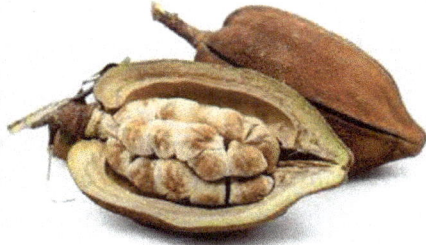

Saba Nut in open Pod

Saba nuts, harvested from the towering Saba trees that can reach up to 40 meters tall, have long been revered for their distinctive flavor profile, often described as a harmonious blend of nutty richness, subtle sweetness, and a hint of earthiness. Their versatility in the kitchen is undeniable, seamlessly transitioning from savory creations to sweet indulgences.

In traditional South American cuisine, Saba nuts grace stews, soups, and desserts, lending their distinctive flavor and texture to these culinary masterpieces. Their rich, nutty undertones enhance the savory notes of these dishes, creating a symphony of flavors that tantalize the palate. The nuts are also ground into a delectable paste, a versatile ingredient that can be used as a spread, a flavor enhancer, or a base for nutritious smoothies.

Beyond their culinary applications, Saba nuts hold a prominent place in traditional medicine. Indigenous cultures have long recognized their potential health benefits, incorporating them into their practices to address a range of ailments, including digestive issues, skin conditions, and respiratory problems. The nuts' rich content of protein, healthy fats, fiber, vitamins, and minerals further contributes to their reputation as a natural remedy.

The Saba nut's cosmetic applications further expand its versatility. Their oil, extracted from the kernels, is known for its moisturizing properties and has been used in soaps, lotions, and other beauty products. Its ability to nourish and protect the skin has earned it a place in traditional skincare practices.

While Saba nuts may not be as well-known as other types of nuts, their unique flavor, nutritional profile, and cultural significance make them a valuable addition to any diet. Their versatility in the kitchen, potential health benefits, and cosmetic applications have solidified their position as a culinary and medicinal gem from the heart of South America. As we continue to explore the wonders of the world's diverse ecosystems, we uncover treasures like the Saba nut, reminding us of the vast array of culinary delights, potential health benefits, and the importance of sustainable practices that preserve these natural treasures for future generations.

Sacha Inchi Nut: An Amazonian Treasure with Culinary and Nutritional Prowess

Emerging from the heart of the Amazon rainforest, a remarkable treasure lies hidden within the Sacha Inchi vine – the Sacha Inchi nut, also known as the "Inca peanut." This nutrient-rich gem, encased in a delicate pod, holds a symphony of flavors, a wealth of nutrients, and a deep-rooted cultural significance that has captivated indigenous communities for centuries.

Sacha Inchi nuts, boasting a mild, nutty flavor and a satisfying crunch, have long been revered for their unique flavor profile, often described as a blend of buttery richness and subtle hints of earthiness. Their versatility in the kitchen is undeniable, seamlessly transitioning from savory creations to sweet indulgences.

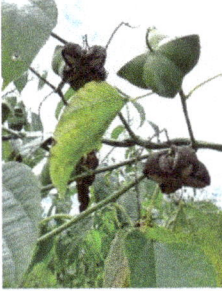

Sacha Inchi Nut on Tree

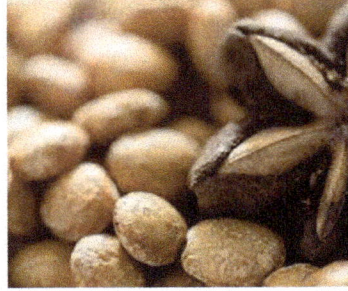

Sacha Inchi Nut in and out of Pod

In traditional South American cuisine, Sacha Inchi nuts grace a variety of dishes, from hearty stews and soups to sweet desserts and snacks. Their rich, nutty undertones enhance the savory notes of stews, while their subtle sweetness elevates the flavors of cakes, pastries, and other confections. Sacha Inchi oil, extracted from the kernels, further extends the nut's culinary reach, serving as a versatile cooking oil, salad dressing, and ingredient in various recipes.

Beyond their culinary applications, Sacha Inchi nuts hold a prominent place in traditional medicine. Indigenous cultures have long recognized their potential health benefits, incorporating them into their practices to address a range of ailments, including inflammation, heart disease, and brain health. The nuts' abundance of omega-3 fatty acids, protein, fiber, vitamins, and minerals further contributes to their reputation as a natural remedy.

The Sacha Inchi nut's nutritional profile makes it a valuable addition to any diet. Its richness in omega-3 fatty acids has been linked to improved heart health, reduced inflammation, and enhanced brain function. Protein, fiber, and essential vitamins and minerals further contribute to overall well-being, supporting various bodily processes and maintaining a healthy balance.

As Sacha Inchi nuts gain international recognition for their unique taste and nutritional benefits, they are finding their way into kitchens and health-conscious diets around the world. Their versatility as a snack, ingredient, and oil is opening doors to new culinary experiences and showcasing the Amazon's rich natural bounty.

Overall, the Sacha Inchi nut stands as a testament to the enduring bounty of nature and the profound connection between humanity and the natural world. Its unique flavor, culinary versatility, and potential health benefits make it a valuable addition to any diet and a reminder of the vast array of culinary delights and potential health benefits that await discovery in the natural world.

Soy nut:

Soy nuts are roasted soybeans that have a texture like that of peanuts. They are a popular snack food and are also used as an ingredient in various recipes.

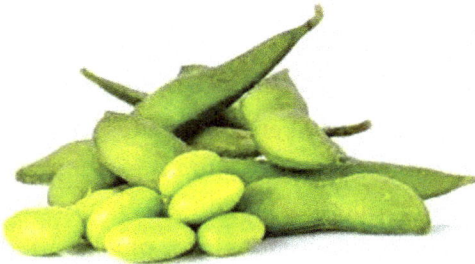

Green Soybean in and out of Pod   Dried Roasted Soy Nut

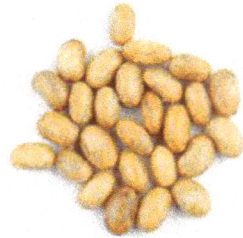

Soy nuts are an excellent source of protein, fiber, and various vitamins and minerals, including iron, calcium, and magnesium. They are also low in saturated fat and cholesterol, making them a healthy alternative to many other types of snack foods.

In addition to their nutritional value, soy nuts have been studied for their potential health benefits. Some research suggests that consuming soy protein may help to lower cholesterol levels, reduce the risk of heart disease, and improve bone density in postmenopausal women.

Soy nuts can be enjoyed as a snack on their own or added to trail mixes, salads, and other recipes. They can also be ground into a powder and used as a substitute for flour in baking.

It's worth noting that while soy nuts are generally considered safe for most people, they may not be suitable for individuals with soy allergies or those taking certain medications. As with any food, it's important to consume soy nuts in moderation as part of a balanced diet.

Tiger Nut: A Small Tuber with a Big Nutritional Punch

Emerging from the depths of warm, fertile soils, the tiger nut, also known as chufa, earth almond, or yellow nut sedge, stands as a small but mighty nutritional gem. This versatile tuber, often mistaken for a nut due to its resemblance to hazelnuts, holds a wealth of nutrients, a unique flavor profile, and a rich cultural heritage that has captivated palates and nourished communities for centuries.

Tiger nuts, despite their name, are not actually nuts but rather edible tubers, similar to potatoes or yams. Their small, wrinkled appearance and distinctive tiger-striped pattern have earned them their name, adding a touch of intrigue to their culinary journey.

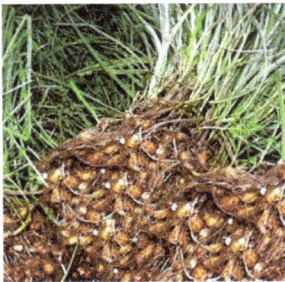

Tiger Nut in the root of Tree   Tiger Nut Harvested

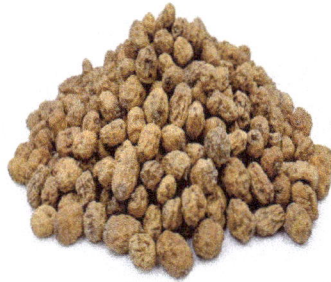

In the realm of nutrition, tiger nuts stand out as a powerhouse of beneficial nutrients. Their abundance of fiber aids in digestion, promotes gut health, and contributes to overall satiety. Vitamins C and

E, along with minerals such as magnesium and potassium, further enhance their nutritional profile, supporting various bodily functions and maintaining a healthy balance.

The tiger nut's flavor profile is as unique as its appearance. Often described as a blend of sweet, nutty, and slightly earthy notes, it seamlessly transitions from savory to sweet culinary creations. Tiger nuts can be eaten raw, their crunchy texture adding a delightful contrast to salads and snacks. When roasted, their sweetness intensifies, making them a delectable treat on their own or as an addition to granola or trail mix.

In traditional cultures, tiger nuts have played a significant role in cuisine. Horchata de chufa, a refreshing beverage made from ground tiger nuts, honey, and spices, is a cherished drink in Spain and other countries. In Africa, tiger nuts are often ground into flour and incorporated into various dishes, adding a unique flavor and texture to stews, soups, and pastries.

Beyond their culinary applications, tiger nuts have a long history of medicinal use. Their high fiber content has been shown to promote digestive health, regulate blood sugar levels, and reduce inflammation. Additionally, their antioxidant properties suggest a role in protecting against oxidative stress and potentially reducing the risk of chronic diseases.

The tiger nut's cultural significance extends beyond its nutritional value and culinary versatility. In many traditional societies, tiger nuts have been used as a symbol of fertility, prosperity, and abundance. They are often incorporated into ceremonies, celebrations, and traditional practices, representing the enduring connection between humanity and the natural world.

Overall, the tiger nut stands as a testament to the remarkable bounty of nature and the profound connection between humanity and the natural world. Its unique flavor, nutritional profile, and cultural significance make it a valuable addition to any diet and a reminder of the vast array of culinary delights and potential health benefits that await discovery in the diverse ecosystems of our planet.

Conclusion

Here are some key health messages regarding nuts:

1. Nuts are nutrient-dense: Nuts are a great source of protein, fiber, healthy fats, vitamins, and minerals. They are also low in carbohydrates and have a low glycemic index, which means they can help stabilize blood sugar levels.

2. Nuts can reduce the risk of chronic diseases: Studies have shown that consuming nuts on a regular basis can help reduce the risk of chronic diseases such as heart disease, diabetes, and certain types of cancer.

3. Nuts can help with weight management: Although nuts are high in calories, research suggests that they can help with weight management. This is likely due to their high protein and fiber content, which can help you feel full and satisfied.

4. Nuts can be a healthy snack option: Nuts are a convenient and portable snack that can help you stay satisfied between meals. They are also a great alternative to less healthy snack options such as chips or candy.

Overall, incorporating nuts into your diet can have numerous health benefits. However, it's important to remember that nuts are high in calories, so it's important to enjoy them in moderation as part of a balanced diet.

Health Benefits of Nuts and Seeds

Nuts and seeds are a nutritious and flavorful addition to any diet. They are a good source of protein, fiber, healthy fats, vitamins, and minerals. Eating nuts and seeds on a regular basis may have a number of health benefits, including:

- **Reduced risk of heart disease:** Studies have shown that people who eat nuts and seeds regularly have a lower risk of heart disease. This is likely due to the fact that nuts and seeds are a good source of healthy fats, which can help lower cholesterol levels.

- **Improved blood sugar control:** Nuts and seeds are a good source of fiber, which can help regulate blood sugar levels. This can be especially beneficial for people with diabetes.

- **Weight management:** Nuts and seeds are a good source of protein and fiber, which can help you feel full and satisfied. This can help you eat less overall and lose weight or maintain a healthy weight.

- **Improved brain health:** Nuts and seeds are a good source of vitamins and minerals that are important for brain health, such as vitamin E and omega-3 fatty acids. Studies have shown that people who eat nuts and seeds regularly have a lower risk of developing dementia and Alzheimer's disease.

How to Eat Nuts and Seeds

There are many ways to enjoy nuts and seeds. They can be eaten on their own, as a snack, or added to a variety of dishes. Here are a few ideas:

- **Snack on nuts and seeds:** Nuts and seeds are a healthy and convenient snack option. Keep a bag of nuts and seeds in your purse or backpack so you can have a healthy snack on hand whenever you're hungry.

- **Add nuts and seeds to salads:** Nuts and seeds can add crunch, flavor, and nutrients to salads. Try adding almonds, pecans, walnuts, or sunflower seeds to your next salad.

- **Use nuts and seeds in baking:** Nuts and seeds can be added to a variety of baked goods, such as cookies, muffins, and bread.

Try adding chopped nuts to your favorite cookie recipe or sprinkling nuts and seeds on top of muffins before baking.

- **Make nut butter:** Nut butter is a healthy and versatile spread that can be used in a variety of ways. Try making your own nut butter at home or buy it from the store. Nut butter can be used on sandwiches, crackers, and fruit.

Overall, nuts and seeds are a nutritious and flavorful food that can be enjoyed as part of a healthy diet.

Recommendations for Enjoying Nuts and Seeds

- **Choose a variety of nuts and seeds:** There are many different types of nuts and seeds, each with its own unique flavor and nutrient profile. Try to include a variety of nuts and seeds in your diet to get the most health benefits.

- **Eat nuts and seeds in moderation:** Nuts and seeds are high in calories, so it's important to eat them in moderation. A handful of nuts or a tablespoon of seeds is a good serving size.

- **Choose nuts and seeds that are raw or roasted:** Avoid nuts and seeds that are salted or sweetened, as these can be unhealthy. If you want to add flavor to your nuts and seeds, try roasting them with spices or herbs.

By following these tips, you can enjoy the many health benefits of nuts and seeds.

Now you know Why and What can send one Nuts.

OOH Yehh Baby!

Join The Nutty Club, Try To Improve Your Health And Longivity.

About the Author

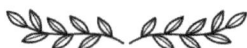

Author Bio: Halsey Cruickshank

Halsey Cruickshank is a remarkable individual whose life's work has been dedicated to health, well-being, and nutrition. Born with a passion for both literature and science, Halsey embarked on a journey that would intertwine these two passions in a profound way.

For over sixty-five years, Halsey has embraced vegetarianism, not just as a dietary choice but as a fundamental aspect of a mindful and conscious lifestyle. This decision has not only shaped his personal health but also inspired countless others to explore the benefits of plant-based diets.

With an unwavering commitment to healthcare, Halsey has spent over 33 years serving as a health professional in private clinics and hospitals, specializing in orthopedic trauma. His expertise and dedication have touched the lives of many, guiding them on their path to recovery and improved physical well-being.

Outside of his professional career, Halsey discovered a unique love and appreciation for a wide variety of nuts. This fascination grew into an exploration of their nutritional value and benefits, leading him to become a self-proclaimed "health nut." He realized that these small powerhouses of nature can play a vital role in achieving a healthy and fulfilling life.

In his debut book, "Going Going Gooone Nuts: A Nutritional Journey for a Healthy Life," Halsey Cruickshank combines his vast experience as a health professional with his personal passion for nuts and nutrition. The book serves as a comprehensive guide for readers seeking to optimize their health through proper nutrition and embracing the bountiful offerings of nature.

"Going Going Gooone Nuts" delves into the science behind nuts, exploring their diverse nutritional profiles and the positive impact they can have on one's overall health. Halsey shares practical advice, delicious recipes, and helpful tips to make nuts an integral part of a balanced diet.

Through this book, Halsey aims to empower readers to take charge of their health, making informed choices that can lead to a long and vibrant life. With a compelling blend of personal anecdotes, scientific research, and practical insights, Halsey Cruickshank's "Going Going Gooone Nuts" is an inspiring read that encourages everyone to embrace a healthier and more fulfilling lifestyle.

www.ingramcontent.com/pod-product-compliance
Lightning Source LLC
Chambersburg PA
CBHW060246030426
42335CB00014B/1615